AMONG WOMEN

Adrian Sangeorzan

AMONG WOMEN

New Meridian

COVER AND BOOK DESIGN by Alexandru Oprescu

LIBRARY OF CONGRESS CATALOGING-IN-PUBLICATION DATA

Among Women
Authored by Adrian Sangeorzan

ISBN: 978-0-997603811
2016946234

Many thanks to Nicholas Kazan who tried to save my voice in translation, to Nava Renek and Alexandra Carides for their editorial work and dedication to my writing. My gratitude goes also to my patients, residents and colleagues at Jamaica Hospital who gave me sources of inspiration for some of the stories in this book.

CONTENTS

INTRODUCTION

IN A TWO-HUNDRED-YEAR OLD French painting, a kneeling gynecologist examines the genitals of a woman who is standing in front of him fully dressed. She is covered head to toe with embarrassment, while he is in formal tails and bow tie. The world has changed since then and shed many inhibitions associated with the profession, although, symbolically speaking, I think it is only fitting that the gynecologist be viewed in this formal way.

I like that Germans call us "Frauenarzt," the ladies' doctor or women's doctor. In other languages "women's doctor" sounds pretentious, even archaic; a medical title removed from the world of exact science, as if what we do doesn't need to be exact and precise. Gynecology comes from the Greek "gynaikos", which means woman and "logos" for science. In other words, the science of women, which sounds even more confused and utterly general, when all that pertains to women, is complicated and miraculous.

At my tenth high school reunion I completely surprised my old school buddy when I told him that I was on my way to becoming a gynecologist. His reaction was sudden:

"You mean you'll be a women's doctor? Why would you do that?"

I didn't know what to say and vaguely tried to explain:

"Perhaps because it's more about life..."

"Very nice" he said. "But how will you ever be intimate with a woman when you'll be doing this day and night, all your life...?"

I shrugged and told him "Never mind", because I liked what I was doing and couldn't conceive that one could be a good woman's doctor if one didn't love women. I used to say, just for kicks, that I've never met an ophthalmologist going blind because of his profession.

I couldn't believe that anyone would seriously ask me why I'd chosen this field so I stopped telling people that I'd chosen gynecology and obstetrics because it was more about life than suffering and illness, and that a woman's universe always seemed more interesting to me and much closer to our human matrix. I knew that perhaps I'd chosen the most delicate of professions because it deals with a woman's most intimate and sensitive parts. Many would have turned up their nose had I said all this. Being still very young, I let my instinct carry me, which, most of the time, is far better than my judgment.

For a number of years, I was completely taken with what I was doing in the hospital, and I didn't even notice that more and more, life around me had begun to deteriorate. I might not have wished to leave my country had not my work as a doctor turned into a game of death and deception. Abortion and contraception were completely forbidden in Romania. The police were closely watching the gynecological clinics and women's hospitals there. Sex had become a risky affair, and women, who carried the burden of reproduction, had reached their limits.

In the mid-eighties, on a dismal autumn day, when the wind blew and dust covered everything, I'd feel as if I was choking and blind to any future for myself. For the next five or six years I kept a low profile, working and living mostly in the Women's Hospital, like a refugee hiding in an embassy, both free and under siege—the embassy of a land where women should have felt protected not harassed and tortured as women were in Romania. They shouldered the hardships and the misery of Communism much more than men and children, those they nurtured and raised as only they best knew how.

For years I secretly worked on different plans for defection. Then the Revolution came. I witnessed it through the Operating and Delivery Rooms' windows. Amidst gunshots, I delivered babies and performed surgery on women and young men who'd been shot in their backs. I had doubts about leaving my country, but after I heard the whisper of bullets going past my ear, I understood that revolutions would not change our world much, nor would they change the state of affairs or that of our people. I told myself that it was better to stick to my plans. I was about to leave at a time when many immigrants were returning, lured and confused by the new type of freedom that was walking the streets with bat in hand and a Kalashnikov on its shoulder. In the beginning, Romania's post-revolutionary enthusiasm caught me as well, but soon I opened my eyes wider.

Some Romanians returning from America told me straight out that I'd be a fool to leave a place where I had everything, just to run away to the unknown and start from scratch. I didn't listen to them. I was a free man at last, the absolute master of the clothes I wore, the passport with the Socialist Republic of Romania seal, and a profession that I clung to as

I would to a life preserver. With a troubled heart I boarded a plane to New York because I'd struck a hard deal with myself. I'd given myself two years to succeed in my profession in the United States. It was either succeed or go back home.

Two months later I found myself in New York, shouldering the gruesome weight of immigration and quickly managed to understand that it's not enough to escape from your cage. I figured out that in the United States there is no shortage of gynecologists, cages, or barbed wire. I ask myself even today what force continued to push me forward since I didn't leave my home country like a desperate man without options or methods for survival.

At the end of the two years, I passed some tough exams and was accepted in an OB-GYN residency program where I had to start my training all over again. After twenty-two years, I'm still at that very first American hospital where I began.

For as long as I remember, instinctively, I wanted to keep moving, to run from one place to another, and I did just that. After reaching New York, a foreign and strange place that I couldn't associate with anything I knew, I didn't have that urge to run anymore. I got seduced by attachment and growing roots in this new land. I felt as if I'd reached the end of the world, and it became clear to me that there was nowhere else to run. Maybe that's why I started to write. Writing would provide my next escape.

Today there are many who, not concerned about my relationship with women, ask me how long I'll keep working at this pace, full time with the hospital, night shifts, plus my private practice? I began to write and publish late in life, only after I felt settled in this new world. After my thoughts and ideas, waves scattered throughout the world, finally caught up with me, I'm at a different station with better reception, better understanding. Besides, I have the chance to live and work in a fabulous city, where all the world that I wanted to know is right here, gathered in one place.

I'm often asked how I find time to read and write. It's as if you lived in the same house with two femme fatales who you equally love and cannot choose one over the other: medicine or literature? I don't think I have to choose… yet!

This is the second book that I've written about my profession. It was written in stages, one story at a time. The first volume: *"Exiled from the Womb, Tales of Woman's Doctor,"* was written from one gasp, an exercise to decompress after years of hardship, insecurity and struggle. New stories and events keep floating around me, and their source remains inexhaustible, as if the women's universe still holds me captive.

As I began to publish, I've been encouraged to continue writing about my experiences as a doctor, where the muse is always "The Woman." It isn't easy to write about what I do, see, and hear daily. Many women might recognize pieces from their own lives in this book. I have to stress that these are just similarities, because all human stories resemble each other. My stories are inspired from situations that I've lived through during my first life in Romania, then in my second one here, in New York. As an immigrant, as a gynecologist caught in between worlds, I still have the feeling that I've lived two different lives, very asymmetrical, intense lives and experiences, which no doubt have changed me, although I can recognize myself as being the very same person.

In the beginning in New York, I filtered everything I saw and did as a doctor through the prism of experiences I'd accumulated in Romania. Now I understand and process my old experiences rather differently. My memories pass through a new lens of understanding. I've found peace with myself, in a place where I had to be reborn, assisting my own delivery, being my own midwife. I learned to listen with a different ear to the stories and dramas of my patients, to those stories found in the new world, also to the ones carried with me, stories which continue to haunt me.

The birth of a child is a rare event, unique to each woman, a special and solid bridge that can connect a doctor to his patients. No woman will forget the experience of giving birth to her child, and the doctor is part of this event. If a doctor isn't touched by this act of helping another being come into the world, it's hard to believe he/she would be a good physician. If somebody would ask me now why I became a women's doctor, this bridge is what I'd talk about, but nobody is asking anymore.

I have many patients for whom I delivered their first, second or third baby; and then I continued to treat them over the years, getting to know their lives, their families, and their problems. I've gotten attached to these people, who continue to keep me tied to this profession.

When I socialize, I'm often introduced to women as a gynecologist, and then I have the chance to listen to their unusual stories and even some unexpected confessions, which sometimes I listen to with some embarrassment. I realize that I'm rather privileged that women relate their experiences to me as a women's doctor. Perhaps they want to use me as a credible witness of some tough events in their lives. This was how I found out that most Romanian women of my generation had their own dramas, whether unwanted pregnancies, dangerous abortions, poorly assisted births, which resulted in serious damage that would be hard to imagine today.

American women are less inhibited and tell their own stories in a different manner. I also have patients who come from the remotest and most isolated places on Earth. They tell me terrible or tender stories, carried with them like stones brought from worlds hard to recognize. Often I have to communicate with them in sign language and eye expressions, which fortunately remain the same everywhere.

A year ago I was passing through Brasov, my old Romanian city where I had worked as a gynecologist for ten years. Everything was different, even the climate. The world I knew didn't exist anymore, except in my head. I wandered like a lost traveler through the medieval city in an almost tropical heat unusual to that place. I got in front of my hospital that looked unchanged, and I was taking pictures of the old walls with the same old cracks I still remembered from before. The courtyard was filled with young women dressed in hospital uniforms and other women of course, some still pregnant, some nursing. A young man in scrubs was smoking and looked curiously at me. He kept his cigarette in his mouth just as I used to do in the days when I used to smoke in that same courtyard.

"Sir, why are you taking photos of this hospital?" He asked in a sour tone.

"Just for sentimental reasons. Do you work here?"

"Yes, I am doing my residency in gynecology and obstetrics."

I don't know what made me ask the young doctor, who suddenly looked like me in a black and white photo taken many years ago in the very same place. "Why did you choose that specialty?"

He was silent for a moment and crushing his cigarette, said: "I'm not sure. Probably because it's mostly about life!"

THE WOMEN'S PAVILION

IF I COULD CHOOSE three things that are important in life, surely one of them would be sleep—such as how to be able to function normally while only getting two to three hours of it. I would live longer and be able to deal with the long "to do" list as I wake up every morning. When the list gets longer, I write it down on a piece of white paper which waits for me by the bedside. If I sleep well, there is a better chance of measuring up. Truth is that sleep was never my forte. Not that I am an insomniac, but when young, I had stretches of time when my sleep was just awful. At that time my future was in front of me, shapeless and dreadful like a crocodile with open jaws ready to swallow me. In the beginning, I was worried, but after I started medical school I began to relax, understanding that my trouble with sleep didn't hinder me when I had to pass a tough exam that winnowed out one out of ten candidates, nor did it prevent me from getting high grades throughout six hard years of medical school.

In spite of those times that turned human lives upside down, the medical profession kept its time honored appearance. White gowns remained respected uniforms, unstained and unblemished, and the Hippocratic Oath was sworn to at the end of each school year just as it has always been. Who else, during those days, could have had such privilege? To pledge another oath than the one we had to pledge to our "beloved leaders". And we pledged it, as if laying a flower wreath at the head of a sick society.

I did my rotation in obstetrics and gynecology in the last year of my medical school in Cluj, right before final exams. At the time I was going through a streak of insomnia that inexplicably overcame me. Everything was seemingly fine in my life. I was becoming a doctor at only twenty-four. I was at the head of my class and had my choice of good places to work, because choice was pegged to grades. I was young, healthy and full of life. Still, it wasn't clear what would become of me after graduation, and mostly what kind of specialty I should pursue. I didn't have a clue, if it would be a surgical or medical one. After graduation we first had to work in the countryside for a year or two, but I didn't want to end up a country doctor in some distant, isolated village. At that time, I hadn't thought of leaving my country and escaping to the wide world like a desperado.

The campus where I was living was a few blocks away from the Women's Pavilion. I was scheduled to do one 'on-call' per week but ended up doing three or four. I couldn't sleep anyhow, so at night I would go to the Women's Pavilion where through the open windows of the delivery rooms, I could hear the screams of the women giving birth there.

The first deliveries I witnessed had a profound effect on me. I had the revelation that I had found what I was searching for. We were living in an upside-down society in which this miracle of coming into the world remained one of the few things that still solidly anchored us to our ancestral reality. Moreover, there was always something going on in the Women's Pavilion, some problem that had to be solved right away, something similar, but also unique, and un-repeatable. My need for action and an adrenalin rush were fully satisfied.

I'll never forget my first 'on-call' shift in the delivery room full of women in labor and busy midwives saying that the full moon was to blame. The warm spring weather had suddenly flooded the city with an unusual hot spell. The windows of the old hospital were wide opened and a warm breeze, laden with pollen and newly awakened insects, swept through the rooms and corridors, blowing away the smell of iodine, formaldehyde and the ancient dampness eroding the walls. The old hospital had been built at the beginning of the Twentieth Century during the Austro Hungarian Empire when Cluj was known as "Little Heidelberg". How proud we were of that! We were sporting custom made purple caps with the college seal, a tradition for our old and "little Heidelberg", but not as mandatory as the hats in our high schools. We still tried to cling to old traditions.

That year, after almost six years of mind bending studying and sheer weariness in Cluj, we became medical school veterans. Now we were the ones who baptized the fall freshmen prom goers, choosing the Prom Queen by measuring the candidates' waist with an old worn ribbon in national colors, and sizing their breasts with some ladles from the Babes-Bolyai University cafeteria. Perhaps half of those six years were spent in the fabled Croco, the coffee shop where medical students gathered in groups, easily recognizable by their thick books and the whiff of iodine and formaldehyde impregnated in their clothes, blended in well with the smells of the coffee shop. After six years the waitresses knew us by name and asked us how long this medical school lasts, for it must have lasted an eternity since we kept passing through that place. After graduation, a chorus of over two hundred newly minted doctors gathered in front of the Croco and serenaded the waitresses with *Gaudeamus Igitur* in four-part harmony as well as with other more intimate songs. When we gave them our prom key, which was another graduation tradition, the waitresses lightheartedly wiped tears from their eyes.

At our twenty-fifth reunion, Croco had become an ordinary bar, with slot machines in the basement and Internet access, filled with truckers and youth sporting tattoos and piercings. The manager was a woman from the old days who told us that old medical students still came by every year like migratory pelicans. She took us down to the bar's cellar where many old wooden keys with the graduation year marked on their ribbons had been deposited.

During our years at the Cluj Medical School there were still some remnants of the old "Little Heidelberg", a shadow of the old fame nurtured with struggle and pride by a few old professors and doctors snubbed and left alone by the regime. Papillian, Goia, Fodor, Preda, the memory of great Hatieganu, were still walking the hospital's corridors and lecture rooms where many generations of doctors had been trained. From the very first year, professors and doctors addressed us as "Mister Student", even though they flunked us at exam time. Our camaraderie was clearly different, because all ailments and diseases are still the same, truly democratic, making us equal.

For that first 'on-call' at the Women's Pavilion, the trees in Cluj had blossomed earlier, and perhaps they were to blame for why so many women went into labor that particular night. When I say labor, I truly say hard labor, and giving birth is awfully hard labor for a woman. Once it begins, there is no going back.

In the old delivery rooms that have remained the same for decades, women gave birth wherever they could on those old delivery tables made in Vienna some seventy or eighty years ago, or directly in their beds. As a student you were not expected to do much. I noticed that one of those women in labor, who was still waiting on a stretcher in the hallway, was about to give birth. She was suffering in silence without letting out the tiniest of cries. During the contractions she would just move her head backwards and arch her back and raise herself on her elbows like a wounded feline. I could see how while she was pushing, the veins of her head and neck were getting engorged, and I had the feeling that something would happen soon. I was just a few feet away when one of the midwives shouted at me:

"Mister Student, come and help."

I got closer to the stretcher where the woman was writhing. When she felt me next to her, she spread her legs wide open. She was thin, muscular, and had the large hands of a peasant who worked the land, with traces of dirt under her nails. She grabbed me firmly by the elbow and squeezed me hard to make sure that I wouldn't leave because she knew that I'd be the only one there when her baby came out. She looked me straight in the eye and softly begged:

"Don't drop my baby, please!"

Then I saw the hairy head of her child ready to come out. It stretched the mother's perineum skin which was wrapped around the baby's head like a pallid crown ready to rip apart. The woman dug her fingers in my arm and was bearing down, pushing for the last time. I had no escape! The baby popped out like a cherry pit, and I instinctively caught it in my arms.

A new born baby is something very slippery and flips like a fish fallen from the sky. It was in my bare hands, and for a few seconds I was stuck not knowing what to do. I was sprayed from head to toe in amniotic fluid and blood. That was my baptism in obstetrics! Before I could figure out what had happened, the woman almost grabbed the baby from my hands.

"Bless you, doctor! A girl, at last! I have four boys at home!"

That was the first time a patient called me "doctor".

The same midwife, in over her head with another delivery, screamed at me through the open door:

"Tie the cord and cut it."

"With what?"

"Use the suture. Put on some gloves first!"

She threw me a bobbin of unsterilized thread that we used to tie umbilical cords. That's when I did the first true surgical knots of my life on that umbilical cord that was still pulsating under my fingers. I clearly felt the pulse of the cord and I waited for a few minutes. There was still blood coming from the mother's side. When the pulse was gone, I did what a surgeon jokingly taught me to do: "Tie it as you'd tie your shoe strings, but tighter and no fold." I was so perplexed that I forgot to cut the umbilical cord, a simple and painless operation. I ran in another room to find a pair of scissors. When I came back, the placenta was out and the woman had already put the baby to her breast.

Later that morning there was only one woman left that hadn't yet given birth. She was pushing with one of the midwives who was as exhausted as the woman in labor, but she kept encouraging her with a tired voice:

"C'mon, mommy. You're the last one. Push hard, I can see the baby's head!"

When she pushed, I could really see the baby's head with its black hair, but it was still somewhere up in the pelvis. Both the woman and the midwife were drained of energy, and the head wouldn't come down. We were all gathered around that woman, and another midwife was trying to push with her elbow from above the woman's pregnant belly. Between contractions they listened to the baby's heart with an old funnel and said that that the heart was "limping." That's how I learned that an unborn baby's heart can "limp."

"Call the doctor!" yelled the Chief Midwife. That's when Doctor Tofan came in. I still remember him today. He was an aging man, well past his retirement, the most elegant man in the city. If he was called from home, he would scrub and get into the operating room still wearing his tie, an old fashioned doctor, who had studied in Vienna before the Second World War. He carefully examined the woman, and I could see how he was slowly frowning while checking the position of the baby's head and the woman's pelvis. Then with the same funnel that had passed from hand to hand all night long, he listened to the heart of that baby who had gotten stuck on his way out and said softly:

"I'm sorry ma'am but it's not working. The baby's head is blocked with its face up, and the heart is skipping badly. We must do a cesarean as soon as possible." The woman happily agreed. She was completely exhausted.

During those days, women were happy to give birth by caesarean section. Its rates were extremely low, only 5-6%. While they were talking, I placed the funnel to my ear and listened to the baby's heart which was low, about 80-90 beats per minute. Meaning limping! I was getting the hang of it, so I helped move the woman into the operating room. Doctor

Tofan did the fastest spinal anesthesia I've ever seen or will ever see, with a long, blunt, needle, twisted and rusted by being eternally re-sterilized in a boiling pot that had its electrical cord patched with duct tape, the needle blunted by hundreds of penetrations through tense spines.

There was no one else around but Dr. Tofan and the scrub nurse Aurelia, a skillful nurse good at all kinds of things. She could continue a procedure on her own if the case required it. The other 'on-call' doctor and the Residents were tied up with another operation.

"Mister Student, would you care to scrub with me?" Dr. Tofan said.

Of course I wanted to be part of it! I started to scrub my hands slowly all the way to the elbows, just as the rules stated, but they screamed at me to hurry up because this was an emergency. I moved to the left side of the patient and Doctor Tofan demanded: "Have you ever scrubbed in for the OR?"

I made a sign that I both had and hadn't. I'd participated a few times at other operations in the Surgical Unit.

"Make sure you don't pass out…" he said while using one fast precise and deep motion to cut the woman's abdomen with a scalpel. Then he enlarged the incision further with his fingers. Nurse Aurelia knew exactly what tools to hand him. I was holding the retractors trying to follow his movements which to me seemed incredibly rapid, almost brutal.

"We must get the child out as quickly as we can," he ordered.

I couldn't figure out when he got into the uterus, which he also opened by spreading the incision with his fingers. He had big, wide, hands, but size is not always an advantage. He tried to get the baby's head out, but he couldn't reach it. It was too low, blocked in the entry or the exit of the pelvis.

"You've got to help me, my boy!" He said in a firm voice.

"Scrub up, open the lady's legs and push the head up." I was lost for a moment.

"C'mon kid, there's no one else to do it."

I got myself under the sterile sheets and placed two fingers inside the woman's vagina where I felt the baby's head blocked, stuck hard like a stone.

"C'mon, push!!"

"I'm afraid that I'll crush the baby's head. I don't think I can, Sir!"

"Yes, you can! There's no 'I can't' here! Push right now, otherwise he'll die! Don't be afraid. The bones in his head are joined and hard. C'mon boy, push it up. Just a little more. OK kid, I feel your fingers. That's it!" I did feel his hand sliding under the baby's head which quickly disappeared as if it was sucked back into mom's belly; in a few seconds it was out in full sight.

The nurses from neonatology quickly brought him back to life, and after a few minutes of resuscitation, the baby began to cry. I was still down on my knees under that surgical table, covered by those bloody sheets as if I were under some holy cloth at confession. I sat there drenched in sweat, blood, and amniotic fluid, full of adrenaline, my heart beating hard.

"Hey, Mister Student, get out from under there! Go and scrub again and come back to finish the job!"

Doctor Tofan let me stitch the muscles, skin, and even tie the knots. The Windsor knot of his tie, slightly sticking out of the surgical gown, remained impeccable, unperturbed by events and changing times, a marker to which one could cling to. I felt that I would climb up his tie like a rope and reach a different planet. At a certain moment he told it to me straight:

"If you like this job, keep your eyes wide open. This profession is to be learned, but its secrets can also be stolen!"

Nurse Aurelia was threading those old eye needles with gut and shoving me the instrument, looking at my tense face. At the end, Dr. Tofan left us alone but not before he gave me a casual tap on my shoulder. Then Aurelia and I dressed the wound and she told me with some tenderness: "Bravo, young doc! I can see that you like to work with your hands. Operating rooms are made for doctors like you."

That morning, for the first time I ate from the patient trays—something all doctors do, having to spend most of their time in the hospital. Then I went back to the dorm. I was still tense, but my head was clear and my heart was light. I walked for a while down the alley lined with trees in blossom, and when I got to my room, I lay down fully dressed straight on the bed and rested the back of my head on my hands, imaging myself somewhere outdoors looking at the sky above. I felt as if I had just finished a long hard day of mowing the lawn. If I had some real grass in my hands, I would have happily chewed some. I fell sound asleep and had a comforting dream. As in most of my dreams I was flying, only this time I was floating much higher and straight ahead.

The next night I was back in the Women's Pavilion. For a long time afterwards, I didn't have sleeping problems.

JUST ANOTHER WEDNESDAY

I HAVE BEEN DOING 24-hour 'on-call' shifts for over thirty-five years. Wherever I would be in this world and in whatever Women's Pavilion I'd be 'on-call' for twenty-four hours, I'd be completely isolated from the rest of the world. Isolated even from the rest of my own life. During those 24 hours, everything else must be set aside. This isolation can be frustrating, but also protective.

Whenever I tried to run away from something, nowhere did I manage to run further and better than inside the hospital I worked in. The Labor and Delivery Room and the Operating Rooms are strangely protective spaces, my space capsule. Doing 'on-call' s for such a long time, I no longer suffer from jetlag. Working nights, sleeping days, or not sleeping at all, I've gotten over the sudden change of time zones, just as I believe astronauts do when circling the Earth at high speed. They go to sleep with the image of Australia and wake up with a view of Europe from up there. We, doctors, whirl about in the same place every day.

Although we have a very static life, when we are 'on-call' the world might just as well be moving around us at high speed. The images we see are changing rapidly while travelling amongst people. After we sign out in the morning, we part saying good night to each other, like soldiers do. There is an almost military spirit in American hospitals, especially in the surgical units, but without that rigid "Yes Sir"/"No Sir". It's some kind of controlled discipline, mixed with the adrenaline rush that those on the front lines have, those who constantly move while facing danger. There are easy 'on-call' days, when I can read or even write, and tough, wild ones, that can tear you apart and turn you upside down by sheer exhaustion and stressfulness. Then you're heading back home driving very carefully, because you're completely drained, your mind is elsewhere, and you don't want to have an accident. At stoplights you may doze off a bit waiting for the green light, but the car behind you jolts you up quickly, since in New York everybody honks if you don't hit the accelerator right away. You get home, eat something, take a shower, and then you don't feel like sleeping just yet.

Sometimes you feel like a soldier back from a dangerous mission, one who realizes that much of what has happened over that crazy night hung together by a thin thread that slipped right through your hands. After such a tough 'on-call' you need some time just to "decompress" before getting back to normal. You think about the women you operated on, by now brought back to life, numbed by morphine, still in the recovery room or the intensive care unit. And these women begin to mix in your tired head with all their bleeding wombs, with all their problems. Finally, you fall asleep with the beeper and cell phone next to you.

There are 'on-call's when the Labor and Delivery (L&D) is like a railroad station, where trains either run late, or all arrive on time and on the same track. In my hospital there are twelve

Delivery Rooms and sometimes they are all chockfull, looking more like waiting rooms, luxurious rooms otherwise, where the TV runs loudly, people eat, drink soda, change the channels and watch games, chat and order Chinese food till midnight, when the fast food restaurants around the hospital close down.

Only the woman, who's there to deliver a baby and around whom everything happens, cannot eat or drink and must stay still in bed connected to all the electronic monitors that we watch carefully from somewhere else. Milan Kundera said that "life always happens somewhere else," but in L&D life happens right there. Unfortunately, we are more connected to these monitors and electronic charts than to the patients in flesh and bone. But at the end we witness life in Prime Time every day. Late in the evening, if we have the chance, we order some Chinese or Indian food and catch our breath in the locker room.

Today, the L&D is no longer the forbidden temple of doom and pain. The hallways are full of people from the neighborhood who move back and forth, and in this strange crowd we, the personnel wearing scrubs, are often in the minority. This is the place where life begins, where you can see daily how fear, worry, and pain mix harmoniously with the greatest moments of joy that human beings can experience. A Delivery Room, with all its monitors, syringes, instruments, personnel and technology is, after all, a corridor of life. If you are not touched by this joy and miracle, you cannot deal with the stress associated with Labor and Delivery and Operating Rooms.

Back in the seventies, when I began to work in Communist Romania, no member of the family was allowed in the Delivery Room. Not even the husband. After he brought his wife in labor, the husband had to go back home where he waited for news from the hospital. Delivery Rooms were like chambers of pain, hermetically sealed.

I was one of the privileged few who participated at the birth of my own daughter, and it was only because I happened to work in the Delivery Room. I had no clue whether she was going to be a boy or a girl, what week of pregnancy my wife was in, when her due date was, or what Rh she had, not to mention other tests that today are routinely done. It was a time when we were completely left in nature's hand, which hadn't forgotten to be good to us. After my daughter was born and I saw that everything was fine, I stayed there and stared at her as if seeing a miracle. Those were long minutes. I was trying to record and remember all her features for fear that she might be switched on us by mistake. She was a miracle and she was all mine!

In America, it wouldn't be a problem if only the husband were in the Delivery Room, or what he's called here, the baby's father. Or the mother. Maybe the mother-in-law, who had to see and supervise everything. When, on top of all the above, there are four or five aunts and just as many cousins, beside some impatient and loud neighbors, the place may become out of control.

By its nature, the soon to be born doesn't want to come on time or at any given hour, so the second and third shift of aunties, cousins and friends have a chance to arrive, new and fresh reinforcements, which only increases the level of apparent disorder and chaos in full swing. When you expect things to take a nice turn just because one or two women delivered and the crowd dissipates happily after the winning game, other women in labor arrive, brought in by their families, by taxi, city ambulances, the police, or JFK airport emergency service, or even by the firefighter's ambulances. It all depends which vehicle gets to the delivering mom first. Wednesday is usually one of the toughest days. Not only because more women go into labor, but because the clinics that serve the hospital send more pregnant women for labor induction. Plus, the private doctors bring in their private patients, knowing that they shouldn't leave for the weekend what can be done in the middle of the week. The indications for labor induction are many and ever increasing, as are those for caesarean sections. Only the ways a woman can give birth to a baby will always remain the same. As we used to say "by below" meaning naturally, or "from above" meaning by cesarean section.

In the USA, mistakes, failures, or "natural" bad outcomes are no longer accepted under any circumstance. We've got to avoid them at any price, even by creating "acceptable" bad outcomes, which at least are within our control.

On one of those Wednesdays the snow was coming down lightly. It was wintertime and cold, but in New York weather can change its mind quickly. By midday the barometer had dropped suddenly, and it began to rain. Then lightning started and some thunder struck rather apocalyptically for a winter's day, but living in New York, we get used to everything. That sudden change in weather put lots of women in labor. Lots of membranes ruptured, water pouring between their legs, pain and bleeding starting, and our Delivery Room was taken by assault.

The Triage, which is like an emergency room where pregnant women were being evaluated, was jammed as was the waiting area where all the chairs were taken. Even the hallways were full of people who accompanied the women. They were coming from everywhere, a kind of invasion. For me, it's quite boring to sit at home in Queens in such weather, because I know that in a Labor & Delivery unit something interesting is always worth seeing. To call the security service and try to send some of these family members home was useless, even reckless, for it could have easily led to a fight.

Otherwise the vast majority of visitors were quiet folk, who respected our work. Some of them were even born in our hospital, which recently celebrated one hundred and ten years of existence since it was first established by some well-organized and kind nuns. Back then, the area we are located in was in full swing, and it still is after a hundred years, although the hospital has been rebuilt a few times from the ground up.

Everybody knows Jamaica Hospital. Twenty-two years ago, arriving from the airport, on my first day in New York, this was the first hospital that I saw because it sits on the very highway that comes in from JFK. It's hard not to notice it when heading to the well-known airport, or if you watch the local channels on TV. This popularity comes because of the many road accidents and other kinds of traumas which continuously feed the hospital's Trauma Center. Or because of news about cops who were shot and brought in. Not to mention some gangster movies in which bandits and cops were riddled with bullets and ended up being taken to Jamaica Hospital. In the last twenty years, it has continued to grow, getting to be one of the largest hospitals in Queens.

Every time I see the TV cameras around the hospital I know that something has happened. That Wednesday was one of those days. When I got into the hospital, the main hallway was heavily guarded by a long line of police officers, dressed in parade uniform, lining both sides of the main entrance.

I thought they were waiting for some known personality to be ushered in safely. Next, a nurse from the recovery room came pushing a wheelchair with a man who had his neck bandaged and immobilized in a rigid collar. He was a neighborhood cop who had been shot a few days ago and survived after the surgical team pulled a few bullets out of him. His colleagues were paying their respect.

Wednesday could have started fine, had one of the doctors from the Psychiatric Unit sent home a patient who not only wasn't well, but was also very angry. Psychiatry as a discipline is very interesting when you read about it, but in practice things are different. That patient, who lived close to the hospital, ran home only to get his fully loaded handgun, then came back determined to shoot the doctor. Only he wasn't allowed to enter the Psychiatric Unit.

It was my 'on-call' day and I already had three cesareans on my list. One of them became, as often happens, an emergency case. The baby's heart rate started to slow down. I turned the woman on both sides, unsuccessfully trying to release the pressure on the umbilical cord. Then, we rushed her to the Operating Room, but the anesthesiologist was nowhere to be found. After a few desperate calls on all the hospital PA system, he phoned back with a troubled voice telling me that he was stuck in the cafeteria and there was no way he could come up.

"Aren't you watching the TV, man? Special Forces are in the hospital and have sealed the cafeteria! I'm stuck here!"

"What Special Forces? What are they doing there?" I asked.

"Just watch the news!"

I immediately turned on a TV which was broadcasting news straight from Jamaica Hospital. The man with the handgun, not finding the psychiatrist, got into the hospital security office and threatened to kill the officers if they didn't find and bring in the psychiatrist right away! I was still connected with the anesthesiologist:

"I'm watching, but what the hell should I do? I've got to deliver this baby immediately!"

"You said that in your country you used to do spinal anesthesia..."

"She's got to be put to sleep, and I don't know how to do that. What should we do?"

"I have no clue. There's a guy armed to the teeth at the door who's saying that nobody leaves..."

I called the Chief anesthesiologist, whom I imagined helplessly shrugging his shoulders. Meanwhile, the baby's heart rate kept falling and recovered only when the midwives asked the woman to position herself on all fours. Clearly there was pressure on the umbilical cord, cutting the blood supply to the baby. I asked her too, contorting myself to the same position, to stand still on her knees for as long as she could. It was a tragic and grotesque scene, and I felt helpless.

To complicate things, she was a Muslim woman from Bangladesh who would only listen to her husband. I have observed that some immigrant women won't dare do anything without asking their husband's permission, even if the permission is asked and given just by a look or small gesture. Her husband was a small and sturdy man, with a long braided beard and a turban on his head. He didn't understand a thing about what was going on and watched the whole spectacle terrified, mechanically translating my orders to his wife. The poor woman tried hard to obey and keep herself in that position.

I've gotten used to working with people from this culture. There are thousands of Bangladeshi around the hospital, quiet people, and almost all of them are named Begum. Even the computers mess up their names and their identity. Being respectful folks, it's easy to get along with them, even when they don't speak English, or they speak something they think is English. All the husbands tell me from the beginning - in a low conspiratorial tone - that they want a woman doctor, but in the end we settle somehow. I used to promise that I wouldn't enter the Delivery Room unless a serious complication arose. And that's exactly what happened that Wednesday. Mr. Begum could not understand why I wasn't doing anything and continued to keep his wife in that grotesque position.

I didn't know what to do while the siege was going on two floors below, but I watched the baby's heart beat on one of the nearby monitors. Thank God his heart was getting stronger. The Special Forces, armed to the teeth, were storming inside the hospital. I ran towards the emergency door, and the first thing I saw was a gun pointed at me. I'd stumbled upon a detective, positioned in between the floors, and he was holding a handgun.

"Sir, I need an anesthesiologist," I yelled. "There's one stuck in the cafeteria."

"Impossible, Doc! An armed man is inside the security room and he's shooting."

Indeed, I heard two gun shots. Who's he shooting at?"

"I have no idea. He's looking for a psychiatrist."

I was glad that I wasn't a psychiatrist and went back to the Operating Room. Mrs. Begum continued to stay on all fours, very tired and trembling, with her head twisted between her arms. That position seemed to keep her baby alive. I exchanged a few looks with the Resident who was going to assist me and with the scrub-nurse who was getting surgical tools ready. They just had empty looks that didn't spell panic yet.

I had two students who were following me like shadows. They were the only genuine Americans around, originally from some quiet American place in the Southwest. They seemed to be the most spooked of all. New York presented itself right there, right now, as it was preached to them on Sundays at their Baptist or Methodist churches, or as they must have seen in some tough movie about this crazy city.

"Doctor! What are you going to do?" asked Mr. Begum, whose face had completely changed its expression and now was flooded with a look of terror that he couldn't hide under his immense beard, or under the turban that covered his face. "Doctor, it's a boy! My first son!"

I pretended I didn't hear that last remark. I knew that in their culture a boy meant far more than a girl, but I couldn't care less about the baby's sex. I just wanted to see that baby out as quickly as possible.

Meanwhile, we heard a couple more shots coming from the floor below. That scene reminded me of my 'on-call' shifts during the days of the Romanian revolution of '89 when I would hear and see night-time shootings happening in front of the hospital. One night, while I was doing some surgery, a bullet passed through the Operating Room window pulling out a chunk of ceiling.

That Wednesday when Thomson, our American anesthesiologist, was kept away by the Special Forces, I was looking rather traumatized at the brand new large, sterile, not expired spinal kit, packed in a huge box full of little instruments with detailed instructions. It took a few good minutes just to open it and lay it on the table. My patient's hands got numb, and she started to tremble harder; then she lay slowly on her side like a wounded animal. The baby's heart rate went down again.

"Ask her to keep the same position," I told her husband.

The woman's knees were trembling, and her hands could hardly hold her. She couldn't stay like that much longer. Her husband said something in Bengali in a harsh tone, or perhaps it sounded harsh to me. It was clear that they communicated differently than I do. Perhaps he told her that he loved her? The woman returned to her miserable position.

We were all watching the TV screen which continued to broadcast live all that was going on in the hospital. A blonde TV commentator, whose hair was blown by the wind, was saying that the Special Forces had entered the hospital and had contained the shooter within the security office. Great! Then another loud gunshot. Maybe the blonde lady on TV had been misinformed? The pregnant woman dropped onto her side again, and the baby's heart dipped to 90 and then 70 heart beats per minute, and wouldn't get back up.

I told the Chief Resident to scrub. Meanwhile I headed towards the emergency exit on our floor where the detective was waiting with his pistol in hand.

"Do you have kids?" I asked him suddenly.

"Why are you asking?"

"In the delivery room there is a baby that needs to be delivered right away. If you don't get me the anesthesiologist who's stuck in the cafeteria, the baby could die. The doctor's name is Thompson. Go get him!"

The detective exchanged some words on his walky-talky then disappeared down the stairs. He was back in two or three minutes bringing Thompson who carried the bag of food he didn't have a chance to finish eating.

"The hell with it. Can't even have a quiet lunch in this hospital. Let's go, man!"

I had known Thompson for a few years. Sometimes he would drive me nuts, but I have to say that he was one of the best anesthesiologists I've ever worked with. A mixed race man from Brooklyn, crazy about music, who'd sing to the patients while he operated on them. He'd always have an iPod with him or a CD player. When I happened to be 'on-call' with him, he would bring his guitar, and if the day was quiet, he'd play the darn thing all night long in the next room. I didn't complain because I too was busy reading and writing. Until the first emergency showed up, a soothing and artistic atmosphere filled the air. I had another colleague who played classical music on the bassoon! The bassoon makes some grave and very bizarre sounds, which can easily make you think of an alarm siren of a boat that is pulling into the harbor. Sometimes he toils for hours on end, making bamboo fittings for that strange instrument, a process that he goes through seven or eight hours a week.

Thompson was single and full of life, a fellow who had a way with the nurses. One day, when I was operating on one of my Romanian patients and he was doing the spinal, Thompson asked the patient what music she'd like to hear. Her husband was right there, and the man asked me rather frightened:

"Is he serious?"

"Play us a 'doina', which is a very melancholic Romanian song that begins with "frunza verde". And he went singing something that resembled Ray Charles, an improvisation that kept repeating "frunsa ferde"!

He couldn't sing anything for Mrs. Begum because he put her fast asleep and intubated her in just a few moves. An urgently performed caesarean section is a very fast operation, even a brutal procedure. At least until the baby is out. Every minute matters. After the skin and fascia incision, everything has to be opened up in a hurry, ripping apart the anatomical layers with your fingers including the peritoneum, the muscles, the uterine wall, until you get to the baby that needs to be saved. Sometimes, all it takes is a minute or two, if you have a good team. The Residents are trained for these emergency caesareans. I remember the stricken face of a surgeon from our hospital that had assisted at such an intervention performed on his own wife. He left the operating room utterly horrified and later told me that the whole procedure looked terrible.

Little boy Begum recovered fast, giving us a few minutes to catch our breath, and then continue the rest of the operation at a more normal pace.

Thompson walked out for a moment and told us that the siege at Jamaica Hospital had officially ended. The guy from the Psychiatric Unit gave himself up and nobody died. In the end, all that came out of it was that he scared to death the guys in the security office and destroyed all the TV monitors until he wasted his bullets. The doctor he was looking for had gone home earlier.

Thompson didn't seem impressed by the whole story. During the surgery, he told us about one of the experiences he had years earlier when he was doing his residency at one of the hospitals in the Bronx. After one of the skirmishes that either the Mafia or the drug dealers have from time to time, the ambulance brought in a guy who was riddled with bullets. Somehow he was lucky enough to have his vital organs left untouched. A bullet passed through his skull but his brain wasn't badly damaged. For ten hours a highly specialized team of surgeons patiently worked to mend and stich his lungs, bowels, kidneys and everything else that was caught in the path of the bullets. Liters of sweat, blood and talent poured out until they got him safely out of the Operating Room. After the surgery, on the way to the intensive care unit, Thompson pushed the stretcher into one of the elevators. Another man walked in just before the doors closed. The guy pulled a gun from his back, screwed in a silencer, and before blowing the brains out of the wounded man, politely told Thompson:

"Doc, pity about all the work done! Good job, anyhow!"

On that Wednesday, as I came out of the Operating Room, I accidently stepped on Mr. Begum's hands. He was praying with two of his brothers, bowing down on his knees right in front of the Operating Room. I apologized and carefully walked around them, avoiding their hands. Then I went down to the cafeteria to grab some food. When we have days like that, we're always hungry. If you are 'on-call' too often, you can put on some weight. We are nervous eaters.

In the main hall there was still chaos. The Special Forces were packing their gear: anti-bullet screens and fiber optic periscopes that let one see from under the doors. Two specially trained dogs were sitting calmly, happy with the outcome. Everything went back to normal in a few minutes as if nothing had ever happened.

A few months later, I was coming back from a trip to Romania and got into a cab at JFK. Mr. Begum, the taxi driver, recognized me right away. He pulled out his wallet, opened it like he'd open a book, and handed it to me through the window divider. Inside was the photo of his first son.

The cafeteria was almost empty. I didn't get a chance to get my food because the phone rang and I had to run to one of the Delivery Rooms for an emergency. A newborn had his shoulders stuck after the head came out. Shoulder dystocia, as it's called, is one of the most frequent complications during vaginal delivery. The baby was probably too large and ate too much while in the uterus, along with his mother. Gestational diabetes which may occur in pregnancy may lead to oversize babies with large shoulders. The head may come out easily, but the large shoulders can get stuck up in the mother's pelvis. It's almost as if somebody opens a door, the main door of life, and sticks his head out only to see that the way out is closing. Then the urgency suddenly escalates and it may become a major drama.

When I worked in Romania I didn't see many shoulder blockages. Towards the end of Communism, the lack of liberty didn't matter as much because freedom is not edible. The food shortage became the major problem, and babies' weights at birth were much lower. America doesn't have such problems. We are living in a world where you only have to stretch your hand, grab food, and put it into your mouth.

Shoulder dystocia happened to the child of a short Mexican woman who was having her fourth birth. The newborn was 'Made in America', with so much food at hand, weighing almost ten pounds. At my arrival, the baby's head was out for a while but was very congested and swollen. The Chief Resident had already unsuccessfully tried all the maneuvers that we knew, but she'd waited too long before she called for help. I was mad at her, but it wasn't the right time to scold her.

In the last two years, due to the larger number of such cases, the administration introduced a new alert system based on codes, norms, and steps that have to be strictly followed. All personnel were trained, through countless tests, drilling sessions, and simulations on dummies. We have to be re-tested every year, starting with students, nurses, Residents and team leaders. It addresses extreme situations like postpartum bleeding, umbilical cord prolapses, or acute fetal hypoxia, emergencies that have to be dealt with right away. The titles and hierarchies may disappear during these trainings. Team work is more important than individual responsibilities. The initiative may not necessarily be taken by the "Chief", but by the one who gets there on time and knows what to do. American hospitals with their emergency units are amongst those organizations that are called 'high reliability' organizations, along with aircraft carriers that have five or six thousand people on board, airport towers and nuclear power stations. American statistics say - and they ought to be believed - that there are still forty-eight thousand people dying every year due to medical errors. Almost as many people died in the Vietnam War.

A few times, while eating in the dining room, I saw how the guys from the Trauma Team responded. They dropped everything and left in a big rush still chewing on their food. When they got to the patient, they knew exactly what to do, step by step, using the fewest words and movements possible. I read somewhere that such a medical team from Los Angeles was sent to train with Ferrari's Formula One racing team, the ones that are able to change a car's tires in six or seven seconds while refueling, checking the engine, and giving the driver a few sips of water.

That Wednesday, looking at the swollen purple head of the newborn, I figured that there was no time to waste. I looked at the hands of the Chief Resident which were a lot smaller than mine. A very important detail! She quickly understood what I wanted and said fearfully:

"I've never done that before! I haven't even seen how it's been done."

I had to get one of the baby's hands out as fast as possible. It was deep inside the mother's uterus. A very difficult procedure, rarely performed. I've only done it three times, myself. For such a maneuver, it's important to have a small hand, but where to get one from? My right hand became wider after I got over forty. That hand had to make its way beyond the baby's head, deep inside the uterus where the baby's shoulders were stuck. I had to find and grab the baby's hand without breaking it and pull it out. If successful, it would result in less of an obstruction from the shoulders that would allow the rest of the baby's body to be delivered. Easy to describe, very difficult to do! Between the compressed body of the baby and the mother's bones there is the tightest space in this world, but somehow my hand had to pass through, otherwise the baby would choke to death. We had a five or six-minute grace period that we'd already consumed. I knew that there might have been some other procedures, all extreme and very traumatic, which nowadays belong to medical history. I hadn't even seen them done back in my old days in Romania: like pushing the baby's head all the way back in the mother's womb, then taking the baby out by caesarean section. It's called the "Zavanneli Maneuver," practiced, I believe, only by Dr. Zavanneli a long time ago in some American hospital in the Midwest. Or, the intentional fracturing of the fetus' clavicle to reduce the diameter of the baby's shoulders. These maneuvers are inconceivable today, although they are mentioned in most obstetrical books. I thought that I'd never be able to reach inside that woman's womb, but desperation pushes you beyond limits and might even shrink your hand a bit.

Somehow I managed to reach the baby's hand, and I then pulled him out into the world. The girl scored weak on the Apgar scale but in a few minutes she recovered and began to cry. One of the girl's hands was swollen and dangling paralyzed, but she fully recovered after one month of therapy.

In the end, the problem was my right hand! It was swollen and hurt. I went down to radiology where I had an X-ray just to find out that one of my bones was cracked. I put a cold patch on and hoped that I would be able to carry on until the morning. For a week my hand was in a cast, and I quickly learned how to do a gynecological examination with my left hand.

Everything would have been fine if six months later I wasn't served with a summons from a large law firm in Manhattan. What had followed after the birth was a typical case of "shoulder dystocia" which happens quite frequently in America. I went through a long trial that lasted five years. I did get to see the little girl playing with her doll while in court in front of the jury. I was acquitted, only after the woman's husband testified that in the end I was the one who'd saved the baby's life. The judge told me that I was "dismissed," which for me meant I was allowed out unharmed, free to walk away grumbling, but with no penalties on my insurance policy, pardoned for doing nothing wrong. "Dismissed" remains a strange word for me.

There was still some time left until I was done with that Wednesday call. We all had the premonition that something else was going to happen. In Romania I heard old doctors and midwives talking about some unwritten "law of the series." Something empirical, of course, which held that when a rare and difficult case shows up, there's a good chance that another one will soon follow. Anyhow, we were already in a state of alert, all pumped up with adrenaline, ready to handle whatever came along. Nobody died, the newborns were all crying at the top of their lungs, everything was fine and under control. Nothing to complain about.

The Chief Resident, a young American lady from a small city in the West, told us half seriously that there was a "jinx" among us. The word "jinx" sounds just as unempirical and medieval as "the law of the series" but nobody cared about this small detail. Still, it was a Wednesday, not a Friday, the thirteenth. Americans have their own superstitions, but in our world of medicine, there's no room for them. The Chief Resident had given birth to a baby girl four months earlier, and every three hours she was "nursing" by attaching her breasts to a mechanical pump. When I first saw her doing it, it shocked me. She was sitting in our lounge almost naked to the waste. On her left shoulder she had a tattoo of the head of a bear that looked quite spooky. During our break, while she fitted the breast pump under her outfit, she pointed to one of the students who'd stuck with our group all day long and said:

"Now I know! He's the jinx. He's been following me since morning telling me that he wants to see some "action". Then she asked me in low voice, "How can we get rid of him?"

I gave the student thirty dollars and asked him to go deep into the cold night and bring us some fresh coffee and donuts. He was an American of Japanese origin, a short man with very gentle manners who spoke strangely in an extremely low and rather grave voice, like those guys who make announcements during professional boxing matches. I was almost too scared to ask him anything. Moreover, he had a kind of eczema on his face, a sort of a rash which became more obvious as the 'on-call' progressed. He seemed happy to witness such a tough night, although he looked scared to death.

He was gone for almost an hour. During that time, a few women delivered back to back as naturally as they could. Our two midwives looked jubilant, ready to prove that as long as they were around, natural births wouldn't disappear. God bless them! We joined the celebration, but our joy didn't last long. The student with the grave voice came back from his dangerous trip, half frozen, with hot coffee, donuts, and a sense of mission accomplished. With him our troubles came back. The Chief Resident also fulfilled her breast milk pumping mission, filling up two little bottles with her own milk, and was in great spirits, ready to jump into action when the hospital's emergency system called us to get ready for another emergency that was on its way to the Women's Pavilion.

When they contact us in advance, it means trouble, and the ambulance brought in a woman who'd been found unconscious in a pool of blood. She lived in a homeless shelter located close to our hospital.

The Physician's Assistant who'd taken care of the Triage area told us that she'd already examined three other women whom she'd put under observation, who had been brought in from that very same shelter. One of the women used to show up once or twice a month to get some food, sleep, and pain killers. She was back that night saying that the shelter was a madhouse where no one could sleep. Our PA had worked in that shelter for a few months and said that the "madhouse" was caused by drug dealers who once in a while brought in cocaine and crack for free, trying to hook up the poor visitors.

The paramedics informed us that the woman they were bringing in didn't have a pulse and they were not sure if she was alive or not. My right hand had gotten a bit swollen, but I could move my fingers, which was good enough. It was past four o'clock in the morning, and the Operating Room had a "double setting", meaning it was ready to handle any kind of delivery. The cardiac defibrillator was taken out from its corner and was being tested.

When they brought the woman in, she was extremely pale but looked alive to me. She could move her hands slowly, couldn't talk, and her eyes were wide open and eager to communicate. I asked her how many months she was into her pregnancy and she showed me eight fingers. How many kids? Any caesareans before? She showed me three fingers. That meant three cesareans! The stretcher was drenched in blood, and the woman was paper-white. Before she was put to sleep in the OR she managed to tell me just one word: "Praevia". A scary word!

The first year Resident intern quickly found her in the data base. Not only had she had a placenta praevia, but it was a total praevia, which sent chills down my spine. The placenta was completely covering the cervix blocking the exit from the uterus. In such a location, the placenta can behave like a strange root that can grow through the uterine wall and even penetrate the urinary bladder. The student with the grave voice and eczema was sent to get blood while the Chief Resident and I scrubbed in a rush. I had to get a larger size glove for my right hand, but I wasn't feeling any pain.

To cut in after three previous caesarean sections, all done through the same incision, feels like you're going through hard cemented tissue, rigid with scars and adhesions. I cut her up and down with small motions, moving little by little into the unknown until I felt something I knew. The first familiar thing I came upon was a loop of small bowel that had adhered to the abdominal wall, the loop held by a tiny hand that had popped out from the ruptured uterus. Those hard adhesions and old scars developed around the uterus were in fact the baby's best chance. The uterus was already ruptured and without that scar tissue the baby would have been expelled into the mother's belly. That would have been a disaster for both the mother and baby.

I cut the uterus in a "classical" way, meaning going with the incision from the bottom up, and I opened it wide as you'd open a book. I managed to get the baby quickly, and he came back to life after three or four minutes. The placenta could not be taken out, nor did I try to because it was "placenta acreta", meaning it had penetrated all the way through the uterus. She was bleeding heavily so I decided to perform a hysterectomy right away. After struggling for more than an hour to remove the uterus, I noticed that the placenta was also "percreta", meaning penetrating through the urinary bladder, a fear of every obstetrician who does caesarians.

In its impetuous process of growing and nurturing the fetus, the placenta can pass through the wall of the uterus and may continue to the urinary bladder which sits very close. The placenta that feeds us as long as we are in the womb can go beyond its range and move further than it has to, spreading danger.

Meanwhile, the rest of the team was pumping lots of blood and plasma into the woman's veins. She'd end up having none of her original blood left. From the lab, we learned that her urine was full of cocaine, but that didn't change the situation. Then out of the blue Thompson announced that the woman had no pulse, and the monitor began to squeal like a broken siren because our patient's heart had stopped. I heard repeated over the overhead speakers "Code 99 at Labor and Delivery" as if we weren't there and couldn't see what was happening.

Everybody was screaming at me to move aside and stop working on the woman who had stopped bleeding completely.

"Boom!" An electric shock sent by the defibrillator almost threw the woman off the table. Nothing on the monitors! Thompson injected a shot of adrenaline right into her heart. "Boom!" a second electric shock that almost passed through me as well. Her life, which didn't get to sneak too far away, came back from a corner of the Operating Room. The straight line and the monotonous squeal of the monitor started to break up, and then a faint bip-bip-bip. The woman's heart began to beat timidly, testing the field, while the blood was gushing again. Blood pouring life. What a great joy! We were back where we started.

I opened the urinary bladder which had been completely penetrated by the placenta. I excised the upper part of the bladder that was bleeding profusely and removed it along with the whole uterus. Then I sutured what was left at the highest speed. I knew well that if the blood, which had been replaced a few times, stopped coagulating, we would be hopelessly assisting at the woman's exsanguination. The whole team was working hard waiting to hear the magic words from me: "We're ready to close."

I'm convinced even today that the woman, the mother of four children, had a very lucky day that Wednesday. A day when her luck touched us as well. Especially in the end when I saw how her urine was turning blue like ink. As I closed her up, I asked Thompson to push some blue methylene into her vein in order to see whether I'd damaged her ureters. The blue urine filling the bag was the proof that we hadn't changed the course of nature too much.

I finally scrubbed out, threw away the gloves and paper gowns soaked in sweat and blood and went to the locker room to clean myself up, but ten minutes later, they called me back on the loudspeakers. Thompson told me that he couldn't extubate the patient because she wouldn't wake up and couldn't breathe spontaneously. She seemed to be in a deep coma. Thompson lifted one of her eyelids and showed me a completely still pupil that had no reaction to light or even touch. That was not a good sign. She was alive though, her heart was beating, but she could have been brain-dead due to the long hypoxia that she'd been through. Thompson asked me to join him and talk to the family waiting in the hallway. Her husband, two kids, a brother, a sister, some people whose accent, or religion I couldn't figure out.

Thompson explained to them that she might not recover and that until she got out of the coma, we wouldn't be able to tell whether her brain had been affected or not. Nobody said a word. Nobody asked a question. Her husband softly said that they wanted to pray. They put their hands together and began mumbling something that was not English. Then they opened their hands and placed them on their heads. I had no clue to whom they were praying. Thompson automatically put his hands together as well and began to mumble some kind of prayer. I tried to do something similar, but my right hand had gotten so swollen that I couldn't join my fingers. I looked at those people in silence trying to remember a prayer I'd heard in my childhood from one of my grandmothers. I couldn't remember much. It was eight o'clock in the morning, the next shift had arrived, and we signed out. Then I walked to the cafeteria with the student with the grave voice and the two Residents. We all smelled badly of sweat and stress. The first year Resident gave me the results of the last blood tests while we were chewing food. We ate quietly and in the end had some coffee. I don't like coffee too sweet and with too much milk, and told them: "Get me a small one. Just a bit of sugar and a drop of blood."

"Did anybody say blood?" someone said softly. They shook their heads, laughing. I asked the student with the grave voice if he still wanted to be an ob-gyn. He didn't say anything. Then I walked in an 'on-call' room, laid down, and fell into a deep sleep. I couldn't pull myself together and go home even though I knew that I couldn't do anything for anybody at the hospital.

When I got up around noon I went back to the Intensive Care Unit. The woman's pupils had begun to respond to light, and she blinked a few times. By evening she came back to life, recognized her husband, her kids, and even myself. Four days later, she walked out on her own two feet.

RESIDENCY IN NEW YORK

LATE AFTER MIDNIGHT it got quiet. All the women who had to give birth had done so. As for those who couldn't make up their minds, the pain had stopped and they were all snoring nicely, numbed by the morphine dripping into their veins. We all got together in the lounge ready to finish the food which was already cold. I still liked the Chinese food and even the damn glutamate they used, which gave me a paradoxical state of exaltation and an almost silly faith in life.

The first year Resident used to order the food brought by a Chinese man who came on the same noisy scooter even when the snow was waist deep. I had learned the menus of a Chinese fast food stand by heart from the very first month of my residency. It was among the many other protocols, drugs and medical abbreviations that we had to grasp. For myself, I would order General Tzo's chicken, and when I got fed up with it, I would alternate to Singapore Mei-fun, some rice noodle mixture that contained all the ingredients that I was completely deprived of in my first life: broccoli, shrimp, baby back ribs, tofu, sesame seeds, lemon grass, etc. Some nights we were so busy that we didn't have time to eat or even go to the bathroom.

With the unusual calm that had taken over the Delivery Room, it seemed that nothing was going to happen until the next shift arrived. What a blessing! We didn't stretch out on the beds because there was still plenty of adrenaline in us to be metabolized, which had accumulated over the day in the form of a strong and toxic ballast, hard to get rid of. I wasn't too talkative at the time because my English was rather crude and limited to the female anatomy, but during that night, after the food and the glutamate had settled in, I began to find my words easier. I was the newest guy on the team, and they were trying to figure me out. They wanted to know who I was, and where I was coming from, who was actually hiding beneath my beard that had given way to its first gray hairs.

Martine, the Chief Resident, a black lady from Brooklyn, had been sniffing around me nervously since I was hired, not knowing how to handle me. I was an intern without "handles", as she would say. I wasn't the typical first year Resident by a long shot, meaning a young man just out of college, idealistic, curious and inexperienced, scared of all that was happening, like a chick that had just come out of its shell. I was scared and anxious, but for different reasons. What terrified me the most was the uncertainty I'd been living in during the first two years of immigration, until I got into that hospital. It was an uncertainty with a lot of inertia I couldn't escape yet, even though I'd gotten to where I wished to be: in an American hospital, in the specialty that I'd been practicing for years.

The first two weeks of residency were the worst, as I was nervously moving around the Operating Room. Martine noticed and told me sarcastically that first I should learn how to do the ordinary chores, like starting an intravenous line, an arterial puncture, dress a wound, and more than anything, to write down intelligible notes in English. She caught me twice writing notes in Romanian during the long night shifts when I was as tired as a dog. After twelve years of practicing in Romania, I felt most at home in the OR. Now I had to poke many veins, write progress notes until my hand got numb, change hundreds of bandages, until I was allowed to put a scalpel or a scissors in my hand. I was coming from a world where doctors, surgeons mostly, were treated like little spoiled gods who would never do "kitchen chores" for the hospital. But here, in America, "kitchen chores" was what we had to start with. Martine told me that my stumbling English did not bother her much; "as long as you do what I tell you, man!" What bothered her was that I didn't know all the professional abbreviations, this being like another language that I had to learn as I moved along. Not to mention learning Spanish.

In that preliminary year, as passing and ephemeral as a first snow, there was also Rego, a Filipino man, a former gynecologist from his far away archipelago. He'd brought over his wife and three children whom he had promised a better life, and they'd finally see with their own eyes that snow truly exists. For them, places with snow seemed to guaranty wellbeing and peace.

Also like us was Shifrin, a former gynecologist from Russia who promised his family that he would bring them to California, where it never snowed. For him, snow and cold meant completely different things. All three of us, with all our experience, were asked to poke veins, write long notes, ask patients lots of details in English, perform dozens of other chores that we were exempted from in the countries, islands, and archipelagos we came from.

Aziz, the Iranian, had been here for a few months. He seemed to be worn out like his Ecco shoes, which he didn't change during the two years we worked together. They'd brought him on foot from Iran.

That night we all sat around eating Chinese food and loosening up a bit.

"And how did you get to Jamaica Hospital of all places?" Martine asked me, looking at me askance, while she was greedily chewing on a chicken wing.

"Two years ago, when I landed in New York, this was the first hospital I saw from the car coming from JFK. I told myself that I would like to be a doctor right here! My wish kind of worked like a professional "imprinting" I said.

I was reading in our medical books about imprinting, a primary instinct in birds. The chicks, which come out of the eggshell, would follow the very first moving thing they saw, identifying it as the mother. In a way, I too was newly born that day when I landed in JFK. It truly was the first hospital I saw, being a few steps away from the airport, very visible from the Van Wick Expressway.

"It can't be true! Were you really dreaming of getting into Jamaica Hospital?"

"It just happened, of course..."

"And what have you done during the two years since you came to America?" They asked me.

I delayed explaining as much as I could. I wasn't going to tell them that I'd been an illegal immigrant with a temporary work permit in the process of being deported. Or, that by carelessly crossing the border into Canada, only hoping to get a better glimpse of Niagara Falls, I got stuck there for over nine months because the American border patrol did not let me come back into the country. Or that later I would be deported from Canada and sent back to Romania, to my old hospital, where pregnancy tests were still being done using frogs, and where my former patients perhaps didn't even notice that I'd left for far-away places.

What would my new colleagues have thought had I told them that in Canada, customs agents pulled me out of a car with a gun pointed at my head, believing that I was some kind of drug dealer? I think it was my medical books filling the trunk that saved me. They were so overused that surely helped illicit mercy from the border guards.

Then, just for kicks, I gave my colleagues a summary resume of Romanian Communism when everything had disappeared like in a macabre trick: food, hospital drugs, syringes, sutures that we used in the OR, rubber gloves, Chinese condoms found in the stores, and last of all, hope.

I told them how we found ourselves with bare fingers in the middle of surgery because gloves were being eternally re-sterilized and would break, and about the rusted spinal anesthesia needles, or about the silk thread which we used when the catgut string disappeared, and other such tricks and improvisations. That's why I didn't like the waste I was witnessing in America where I could see tons of packaged material thrown around the hospital. Three gloves used at one time, one pulled on top of the other, instruments for laparoscopy yanked out of their boxes and tossed around without being used. Everything had a one-time use, except for us, mercilessly used and reused a hundred hours a week.

Martine, licking her fingers covered in duck sauce, told me: "'Imprinting,' you said, eh? Well then, I'll be your 'mother hen' this year, so keep following me around! And loosen up for God's sake. Nobody's going to eat you alive!"

Martine was indeed a good mother hen. She walked like Donald Duck. The only thing that I had to do was keep at a certain distance when she spoke because when she stressed the words so I could understand her Brooklyn accent, she sprayed me with saliva. The Chief Resident in an American hospital has lots of power. It's like a front-line army sergeant during a time of war. A Chief Resident could do to you whatever she pleased, and if you didn't do your job well, you were a dead man.

After a few weeks I was part of the team and everybody let me be. During quiet nights, I could even take a short nap. Later, on one of those nights, one of the nurses, a Filipino lady with an angelic face, stormed into the room where I'd fallen into a deep sleep and dragged me out of bed.

"Doc, come quick! She's giving birth! It's a breech!"

Years later I kept remembering that night. By then I'd been working with this nurse for almost twenty years and she had often gotten me out of the 'on-call' room in the middle of the night in the event of a great emergency. It was towards the morning, and I knew that the delivery room was empty, and yet I heard the woman who was about to give birth screaming at the top of her lungs. It was a breech! Lucky me! Not long before, I'd just been telling them how in Romania, we delivered babies who were coming feet first. In the U.S., the only way breech presentations were allowed to deliver vaginally was if the woman arrived at the hospital at the very last moment and there was nothing else to do.

I grabbed a pair of gloves, put them on, and rushed into the delivery room. The woman was screaming like crazy and was already on the table. I tried to examine her, but I couldn't because she was still wearing clothes. The nurses and the other interns were watching silently from the sides.

"C'mon, help her get undressed!"

But the woman was extremely agitated, kicking and screaming.

"Let's go, momma, take it easy. Let me help you get undressed." I raised my voice a bit to quiet her down because she was kicking me. It may happen that a woman can get into an uncontrollable state during delivery, when she can hurt herself or her own baby by mistake. I had been involuntary kicked a few times, scratched, and once in Romania, I was even bitten by a fourteen-year-old girl who jumped up from the obstetric table and hid under the table while she gave birth. She bit my hand instead of biting the midwife who did not want to give her a pain killer, "just to teach her a lesson."

Usually, when I can't control a woman in labor, I make eye contact with her, grab her hand, and try to talk to her. That night no one else was moving a finger, and I couldn't do anything with that woman regardless of how hard I tried. When she couldn't hold back her laughter anymore, she revealed her face. It was Chief Martine who'd stuffed a few pillows under her clothes pretending to be pregnant. All the other Residents were rolling with laughter and pointing to the calendar on the wall.

"Doc, it's April Fool's Day!"

I had no clue that they were keeping with tradition.

"C'mon, learn how to laugh, man!" blasted Martine, while the others were brought to tears.

Beginning that day, I took their advice and loosened up a bit.

The story of Aziz, the Iranian intern, was a lot more frightening than mine. When he told us how he'd escaped from Iran, everybody was scared stiff. It made me realize how little I knew about the rest of the forgotten world. I thought that my old world and experiences were at the bottom of human existence!

Aziz had escaped from Iran through a smuggling network that specialized in human trafficking. Desperate people, truly desperate. Two of his brothers had been killed in the Iraq War. In exchange for a sum of money put together by his family, he was placed into the hands of that clandestine network and had to cross mountains in Iran by foot, reaching Turkey in two weeks. Before he left, his sister bought him a pair of sturdy Ecco shoes, to make sure that he wouldn't get to America barefoot. By the third year of my internship, I too bought a similar pair, even though I didn't have to run away anymore. Of the group of fifteen that left Iran, only eight made it to their destination. The rest mysteriously disappeared forever, killed on their way either by their "guides" or by bandits.

Each one had a password which they had to give at the very end of their journey. I don't exactly remember Aziz's password, but like any secret password, one had to say it only when it needed to be revealed. The ones who said it too early were either killed or robbed. They slept during the day and traveled from place to place during the night, dropped by some traffickers and picked up by others. His family found out that he was still alive only after he reached New York. He also had been a gynecologist in Iran, where in the neonatology ward they used to cover baby girls' little faces with veils from the very first day of their existence.

In the following years I worked with a few other passing interns from Africa, Vietnam, India, China, Burma, Haiti, and I understood that the hard times of Romanian Communism were just a nice story compared to some of the nightmares the other folks had endured.

Rego, the Filipino, was one of the cheeriest of all the people I knew. During the Marcos dictatorship, his father and older brother had been executed in their courtyard in front of the whole family. He didn't lose his perpetual smile but swore that he'd go to America or another place that had democracy and snow. I don't know why he believed it, but for him snow guaranteed peace, freedom and good life. Like myself, he was already an experienced gynecologist but we had to start from scratch. We were all doing the so called "preliminary year," and when hired, were clearly told that in a year we'd have to leave the program and find something else. Nobody would have accepted us in any residency program without this "American experience." In the end I think they were right.

After a few more months, another guy came on board, Hesham, an Egyptian from Alexandria, who looked like my twin pharaoh brother. We were of the same age and we shared a similar professional past. At least I believed so. When we had a difficult case, it was enough to only look at each other in order to communicate. We figured out that once we would be integrated into the American system, we foreigners, with all our past experience, could be quite valuable assets to an American hospital. At the beginning we functioned mostly as interns, or, as they referred to us, "house officers." We were called "officers," but we were just first line soldiers, good at everything from small chores to difficult operations. In the OR we could easily take over complicated procedures because we had more surgical experience than some young ob-gyn Attendings. It wasn't simple to deal with us, and our Chiefs didn't exactly know how to treat us. We learned to bow our heads, and we did exactly what the Chairman asked us to do: "keep a low profile." We worked hard for little money, hoping that at the end of the year at least one of us would be promoted into a Resident position. We knew well that there were others just like us waiting in line, desperate and hungry.

Hesham had worked in a large Egyptian hospital, one full of shortcomings and problems, like mine in Romania. In Egypt, he was left alone and allowed to work by himself, after relatively little training. He'd seen cases one would rarely see today, and he had to solve them somehow. To his advantage, in his former hospital, he had a simple laparoscopic kit Americans designed just to sterilize women. Using it daily, he learned how to do other complicated procedures. Today, he is one of the best laparoscopic specialists in New York.

He too had a tough immigration story to tell. Hesham came to America with a small suitcase, his medical diploma, and two thousand dollars in his pocket, convinced that this money would be enough for a couple of years. He told me how he was commuting daily from Staten Island where he was living with a cousin from Cairo who'd told him that the Staten Island was close to everything in New York. Hesham's trips took three to four hours each day, walking to the bus station, and then taking the bus to the ferry terminal where he'd board a boat to Manhattan. Every day the ferry passed the Statue of Liberty, the main reason he'd come to the U.S.A., but which he only noticed on a bright sunny morning after five months of commuting, when he finally raised his eyes from the ferry's dirty floor.

We learned that people in America "do observe" important events, such as Christmas, Hanukah or Ramadan; meaning that some "celebrate", while others "observe", so we all could enjoy them. During those days, all that we could "observe" in life was what could be seen between the legs of the women who gave birth at Jamaica Hospital, or the ones we examined in the clinics. For quite some time, our private lives disappeared completely.

On another quiet 'on-call' night, he spoke freely and told us a story that baffled us all. When Chief Martine, a hard core American, asked him why he'd left his country, which she believed was somewhere in Europe, Hesham plainly said that he left his motherland because of cats! We thought the man was going nuts; after all, it wasn't hard to lose your mind during the Residency. We were just having our Chinese food, and Martine suddenly stopped eating:

"Cats? Were you a veterinarian in your country?"

"I am talking about the women's hospital where I worked many years," Hesham said. There were hundreds of cats roaming around in the hospital, in the crowded rooms, between patients, in the hallways. Everywhere you looked, you'd see a cat waiting for a morsel. Nowhere else in Alexandria were there so many cats. I can see them right now in front of my eyes."

We looked at him concerned.

"Are cats holy in Egypt?" I asked, thinking of the old statues from ancient Egypt amongst which I knew to be some carved cats and dogs. Perhaps it was like in India where cows are holy, and roam freely through the cities without being hurt.

"Not a bit! There were so many cats because human placentas were tossed into the hospital garbage bins and were quickly eaten. That made the cats breed fast and thrive."

In that moment we all stopped eating. Only Hesham kept swallowing, not at all bothered by the memory of cats greedily eating placentas.

In my Romanian hospital, placentas were placed into a large freezer and once a week hauled to the Nivea factory in the city. Because of their high content of hormones and nutrients, they were used to make expensive facial creams.

Some of the older midwives were still using them to collect "vernix caseosa," that natural cream that covers the newborn's skin, yet another residual product of birth. Sometimes this cream is so abundant on babies' bodies that large chunks are left on the operatory sheets after the babies are extracted through caesareans. I liked to challenge new students, always emotional, and ask them what they thought the white cream was. One of them answered with a straight face that he thought it was chewing gum—a well chewed piece, because it looked exactly like that. In the olden days, midwives collected this cream and would sell it to princesses and rich ladies for a dear penny. Anyhow, the expelled placenta, also called "the baby's house," remains a useless and redundant tissue after birth, with an almost extraterrestrial look. In Hesham's city, its cosmetic value had not yet been discovered, so it had been fed to cats. Dozens of placentas every day.

"I hated cats," continued Hesham while eating, "but we got used to them. There would always be a cat jumping around when we least expected it. Once a year a gunman was hired and with a BB gun, hunted them mercilessly throughout the whole hospital. He would gather a big mound of dead cats in the back of the hospital, but they came back in no time. One day I did a hysterectomy. After I removed the uterus, I placed it in a jar to send to pathology to be sure it was not cancerous. I never got to know, because a big tomcat came in and disappeared through the window with the uterus. That was the day I decided to leave my country."

Disgusted, Martine wiped her hands with a hospital napkin, shoved the food aside and said: "You guys, are sometimes too much! Back to work!"

We were always back to work. Had I known what Residency in America meant, maybe I wouldn't have emigrated, and I'd still be in my Transylvanian city where I'd made a good name for myself, had lots of nice patients, and there were no cats in the hospital. I immigrated when I was thirty-six, after the fall of Communism, when , full of gunshots and street fighting which I saw from the hospital window where I was stuck for two days and two nights amongst the wounded and dead. Women kept coming to give birth, even at that historical crossroad.

I got to America with a suitcase and two hundred dollars in my pocket, which I knew wouldn't last too long. I began my Residency in New York, exhausted and squeezed like a lemon, after two terrible years of immigration. I finished it at the age of forty-two, ready to start all over again, with a surreal determination that only comes out of the ashes. Today, I still work at the same hospital. Tens or hundreds of Residents, Interns, students and Attendings have passed by. Now I'm the veteran of that Women's Pavilion.

Male doctors in gynecology are on the way to becoming extinct. The main reason is that women want to be examined by women, and many men do not accept that their wives, girlfriends, and daughters, will be examined by another man. There is no American law to protect the rights of men, although it seems that federal funds cannot be used for any kind of gender discrimination. A colleague from Connecticut had to close his office after two young female doctors freshly out of their Residency opened their office in his little town. My colleague went bankrupt and had a hard time finding employment elsewhere. He even wanted to sue the American government for gender discrimination. Of course nobody took him seriously.

The truth is that in obstetrics and gynecology, women are more easily accepted in a Residency program, and after graduation find employment much quicker and are better paid. Of the fourteen interns we have in our program, only three are men. It seems we are a specialty that is slowly going back to a matriarchy, that type of ancient society when women were leaders, pulled the strings, and kept the world at their bosom. There were no wars, nor was there a rigid hierarchy in those societies. Let it be!

Almost all of the 'house officers' in those days were former gynecologists in their countries. They had eventually succeeded in finishing their Residencies, even if they had to do it all over again, in four, five or seven years. All except Rego, the Filipino, who after three years of hard work and snowless winters, took his family and disappointedly returned to his country.

We had yet another outstanding house officer, Monique, a Swiss woman born to a Swiss father and a Taiwanese mother. She spoke six languages fluently, including Mandarin. She'd lived all her life in Switzerland where she'd gone to medical school. We often asked ourselves what the hell was she doing in a tough place like this: a fine woman like her, educated, wealthy, with a promising future in Switzerland! She'd even completed a year of surgical training in Bogota, Colombia. Rarely did I see a more dedicated doctor in our profession, with such talent for surgery as Monique had. Not finding a position as a Resident in a hospital, she went back to Zurich University. It seems strange and hard to believe that a Swiss woman had to go back to the foothills of the European Alps deeply disappointed. In Queens, she lived in a pitiful neighborhood, full of immigrants, close to the hospital, and would come to work on foot because her car was stolen twice. When her troubled year was over and she had to go back to Switzerland, she cried. I couldn't help but ask her why she cried like that.

"I don't know, but this crazy city fits me so well."

A year later when new opportunities opened for foreigners, because our specialty started to be less desired by American graduates, I tried in vain to get in touch with her and Rego, just to bring them back. They'd loved New York and got along well here, but had burned all their bridges to the New World.

Residency is the toughest time during a doctor's life. I could compare it with the life of a Marine during Boot Camp training, only it doesn't last three months but four to five years. It has some of the toughness and rigorous demands in order to form an officer for the frontline. During Residency you spend your life dressed in scrubs stained with blood and heavy sweat, uniforms with no rank. The hospital is the garrison that one rarely leaves during those years, only to get some sleep, eat, read a few medical books, and keep minimum contact with the ones around: with family or a partner who would wait more or less patiently for the end of your ordeal. You don't need many clothes or shoes because there's no time to wear them. As much as I tried during those four years, I couldn't wear out a set of clothes or a pair of shoes.

For nine months I belonged to a Residency program from Long Island which had not been affiliated with the CIR, a kind of union for Interns and Residents. That's why we had to put in one hundred and ten hours a week or even more. Not less, but not more either. "Keep a low profile. Yes, Sir! Sure, back to another hospital's kitchen chores." I was forty, and again a first year freshman. I wasn't missing veins anymore, and I was writing down notes correctly, starting at five o'clock in the morning. We were not allowed to come in earlier, and when I began to show up at four or four thirty, the Chairman called me in and told me to show up when I had to, at five o'clock sharp.

"Why not earlier, Sir?"

"Because that's the rule, doc! If you go over 110 hours and you break down, the hospital doesn't want to be taken to court by the family."

In my case the risks were obviously higher. I was so tired that I began to have all kinds of fantasies, starting around four a.m. when the alarm clock rang. I was thinking that it wouldn't be bad to be hit by a car while crossing the road. Then one of my legs would be put in a cast and I'd get some rest for a while. But only lawn mowers and squirrels crossed the hospital grounds.

Carmen, a third year Resident, a hardworking Puerto Rican with a constant smile, told me that she too had dreams about being in a leg cast, but that she'd gotten over it. We worked side by side from early morning till late at night.

I wasn't hit by a car, but in the end something did happen to me. I was forty and trying to stay in shape. I began to exercise during the short breaks we took. I was coming to work at five a.m. sharp. Then I would go through the whole obstetrical ward, patient by patient until seven o'clock when I could have a coffee break. Finally, I got into the Operating Room where I felt rather protected. Carmen was puking everything she ate because she was pregnant. I would give her an intravenous with fluids and vitamins, and then I would exercise for twenty minutes, walking up and down the stairs of the twelve-floor hospital, or do some squats and push-ups.

One day, while I was scrubbing for surgery I looked at myself in the mirror and saw that I had a bump right over my right collar bone. It wasn't painful and that worried me most. Being a doctor, I knew that what hurts from the beginning couldn't be cancer. I wished I was in pain. Just as I came out of the OR I showed my bump to Pandhi, the Chief Resident, an Indian from Calcutta, who was so impatient to finish his Residency that he didn't care about anything else.

"It's suspicious," he said dryly.

The biopsy I had was also suspicious, and my knees went weak. Weak and trembling knees, plus the sensation from a dizzy head and empty stomach, through which the bats of fear started flying, becomes a very counterproductive state for a Resident who must work 110 hours a week. I went to see our Chairman and told him that I needed to have surgery as soon as possible.

They scheduled me for surgery at five p.m. that Friday, the last case of the day. Up to that moment, I worked in the Delivery Room with a troubled look on my face, which didn't go unnoticed by the nurses. Even patients asked me: "are you OK, doc?" I didn't have lunch, because surgery had to be done on an empty stomach and at 5:00 pm I laid down on the operating table. They put me to sleep, and I woke up an hour later with a huge bandage over my collar bone and with my right hand immobilized. I looked as if I was freshly hit by a car on a crossroad. I was discharged with clear instructions: "You keep it this way for two days; get some pain killers over the weekend, and Monday at five a.m. get back to work, doc!"

It wasn't easy to talk to Pandhi because I knew that he wasn't knowledgeable about this type of lump. Besides, he was rather too direct with what was crossing his mind. I was also afraid that being a Hindu, he would start talking about

Karma and the benefits of being reincarnated into some better and easier life, let's say a dermatologist. I had been working with him for three straight months of night shifts and often he would say with sadness and melancholy: "Why in hell didn't we become dermatologists?"

"Pandhi, leave it for the next life!" I'd respond.

During that unexpected free weekend, I was seriously thinking about the kind of life I was living, about all those years of torment, troubles and the crap I'd endured. I didn't regret anything. Only, I wasn't rushing to be reincarnated. I went back to the campus, into my studio, and when alone, I was overwhelmed by thoughts from our gentle Eastern Orthodoxy, whispering something like: "That's life, doc! You were fretting like hell and in the end you're hit not by a car, but by a damn sarcoma that might free you forever. Amen!"

I tried to call Sandu, one of the hospital's three Romanian Residents doing internal medicine, but I changed my mind. The man had gone through real hell in the last few months, and I thought he might not need an existential conversation. He came from northern Romania, a region called Moldova, and spoke with a sweet and mellow accent. We called him "Oleaca"—meaning in Romanian "just a little bit"—because for him everything was neither too much, nor too little, but just "oleaca", like he said.

We had just "oleaca"—a little bit—until our Residency was over, and twice that much until we'd become real doctors in America. Sandu's wife, also a Resident at a hospital in Manhattan, had another notion of time and space and wasn't able to handle the hell we all were going through. For a few months Sandu and I commuted daily to Manhattan. We were so tired that when we drove our cars, we would be afraid of falling asleep behind the wheel. One of the Residents who commuted to New Jersey died a year earlier in a terrible accident. While he was driving to work, he just fell asleep. That's when they enforced the 110-hour maximum rule.

When I was extremely tired, I used to push a finger against my forehead right between my eyes. I'd discovered the trick by chance during a multiple choice exam lasting three hours with no breaks. Each little break could cost you a few questions. When I got home after one of those exams, I noticed a small wound right between my eyes. Pandhi explained it simply:

"Why do you think that we, Indians, mark that spot with a red dot?"

I taught Sandu how to help himself and stay awake at the wheel when he went home tired. A few months back, when we were both working nights in the ER, his name was called on the loudspeaker. I saw him drop the phone, paper-white, and he left in the middle of the night without saying a word.

He'd just found out that his wife had thrown herself through a window from the twentieth floor and had been found dead on the sidewalk. When he came back, he told me in few words about the depression his wife couldn't deal with. For a while he was saying that he would give up on everything and go back to Romania. It turned out that he did manage to finish his Residency, marry a Russian nurse, and leave for France. I don't know what became of him, just like I know nothing else about many other doctors with whom I've worked. Some came out of Residency completely broken-up, some never finished, others got hooked on drugs and booze. Residency is not a normal state of mind!

Because of my surgery I ended up with a free weekend, enough time to deeply contemplate the possibility of shifting to a "lighter" specialty. I spent those days with a couple of close friends. One of them, a passionate photographer, had taken my picture three months before while I was sleeping on the shores of a lake, collapsed after one of my 'on-call's.' It was he who diagnosed me. When he took the shots, I had no bump above my collar bone; it could have been easily seen because I'd lost a lot of weight. No cancer can grow that fast. When I went back to the hospital on Monday, I tried to extend my leave because my hand and my shoulder were still swollen. I called Pathology and they told me that there was no cancer. The Chairman advised me to take it easy with my exercise. The next hour, I was scrubbing for a caesarean section, and, as hurt as I was, I was happy to continue my residency in Gynecology.

In Romania, where I did my first Ob–Gyn Residency during the eighties, only doctors under thirty-five were accepted for surgical specialties. Administrators believed it wasn't worth investing in a doctor over that age. In America there are no age limits for doctors, just as there are no limits to anything. This fantastic "advantage" can finish you off. I came out of Residency fine, probably because of my stubbornness and desperation. When I left Romania, I had made a deal with myself: two years to make it, or go back to my old life in my old hospital. I had already invested twelve years in this specialty, which had become my life. I had to do my entire Residency all over again in New York. Residency in America was indeed my greatest test of endurance. Along with all the immigration stress, it was a very toxic mixture, against which I slowly learned how to protect myself. However, had the stress not eased-up over time, it would have finished me off.

When I became Chief Resident, the Chairman asked me to interview an atypical American graduate.

"Tell me what you think. You might work with him every day!" In the end the professor added smiling: "Try to be kind! He's older than you..."

Before the interview, I found out that the man had been kicked out of a very demanding Residency program, affiliated with one of the great universities.

I came face to face with a six foot six guy, well built, visibly older than me. He wore large glasses that made his blue eyes even bigger, but his eyes convinced me that he deserved another chance. Those were the eyes of a man who could not lie. I asked him a few tricky questions, strictly related to hospital business, using plenty of medical abbreviations and short expressions just to test him. He had large and strong hands, full of callouses like those of a carpenter. Looking at his huge hands, I was thinking of the poor women—our patients, but I knew that our profession does not rely on hands alone.

His name was Lermontov, and the first thing he told me was that he was not related to the great Russian poet. He spoke clean, precise English, as if he was an educated TV anchor, dryly presenting some simple news. He was born in the U.S. but spoke good Russian, only he could not read it. To speak Russian is a big advantage in my hospital because there are many Russians in Queens. Lermontov was a strange mix of a straight civilized American, with a well-hidden savageness, which attracted me from the beginning. A weird human cocktail, entirely different from what one could find amongst the Eastern Europeans with whom I was related. I asked him directly why he'd gotten kicked out of his previous program. He answered candidly, with an almost childish face: "I don't exactly know why... The Program Director didn't like me from the beginning. I was put on probation after I wrongly administered a dose of Heparin. Nothing happened to that patient. I discovered my mistake on time, but after a second blunder, he didn't renew my contract. He just said that I was too bohemian to be a doctor..."

His remark brought a strange smile to my face, remembering that I myself had been accused of being too "bohemian." During the eighties, when I was a young promising gynecologist, my former boss in Romania, a good doctor and good man, kept pushing me to join the Communist Party. "Otherwise you won't advance hierarchically and lots of little people will walk all over you."

One day he asked me to help the party secretary in the Operating Room. She was also a doctor, an ageing woman who'd forgotten how to do surgery as she'd forgotten female anatomy. She just wanted to make a buck. That day, during a difficult caesarean section, she thought that the patient's ovaries were unusually large as they should be during pregnancy. She wanted to remove them. In vain I tried to stop her, explaining first, then getting really mad, yelling at her, throwing off my gloves in protest and furiously scrubbing out. She castrated that poor woman with a few precise movements. It is so easy to remove a woman's ovaries. Comrade Secretary had learned to do that very fast.

"You are such a damn bohemian," she said, even after the pathology had shown that she pulled out two normal ovaries.

"What are you fretting about?" she continued. "This woman has four kids; she doesn't need her ovaries anymore."

That's how I lost my last chance to join the Communist Party—by being declared an incorrigible bohemian. Though I liked to be viewed that way. I was reading quite a lot, toying with poetry, listening to good music, but I reached the peak of my bohemianism only when I decided to tell them good-bye and leave the country.

"How long haven't you worked?" I asked Lermontov.

"It's been two years."

"What did you do in the meantime?"

"I try to travel; built a small bungalow in the woods... I continued to read medical books because I like them. I had an extra chance to ponder the overall meaning of my life..."

No comment. The man seemed bohemian and sincere, almost masochistically sincere. Lying is harshly punished in America, but not the bravery and claims of overachievement, which are highly encouraged from kindergarten. Children have to grow up in America with a huge dose of self-esteem that has to rise sky high, no matter what. When they hit the harsh reality of life, they don't know what to do and end up going to a therapist or taking drugs. Modesty and humility, which our parents and teachers served us spread on bread, is not taught in American schools. In the States, it's inconceivable to accept our old Romanian saying: "the sword wouldn't cut a bowing head," a saying that has been drilled into each generation, to the point of being constitutional. Here was the American Lermontov, a man who never bowed his head, with noble pride, discreet and sad, even endearing. Although he might have taken plenty of blows before and his future seemed seriously threatened, he still kept his posture with dignity, even though in his blue eyes, one could read desperation, seemingly appeased, but still desperation.

Lermontov was in a far worse situation than I'd been four-five years before, when I desperately needed a job, any job. In the last two years, nobody had given him a chance. He was an American graduate with over $200,000 of debt accumulated over six years. He graduated from medical school when he was forty, and now he was forty-five. A strange American, a descendant of a family of Russian nobles who'd taken refuge in America after the First World War. He was the nephew of a white officer three times sentenced to death and who managed to escaped each time. Lermontov remained a somber yet eternally smiling man, even though he was more desperate than many of the immigrants with whom I'd been working. He had three grown children, was a grandfather of four, and for over three years he'd been living with his wife on some large boat which he pompously called a yacht. He arrived for the interview by sailing his boat down the Hudson River all the way from Albany.

I gave the Chairman a good report, and he hired Lermontov on the spot, just like he had done with me. He just said: "Keep an eye on him. Let me know if something goes wrong!"

For the next four years we worked together day after day. Even though he had giant hands, he managed just fine with women. No one complained. His judgments were right most of the time, and he quickly learned how to use his hands in the Operating Room. He was never ashamed to say "I don't know" when he didn't know something – and I always appreciated that.

The boat he has been living on was tiny, and it was kept in the Glen Cove Marina where it was hooked up to water and electricity, but those were his only connections to the rest of civilization. Also living on the boat was his wife, a nurse in the Bronx, and a claustrophobic cat that slept up on the mast during the summer months.

Every day, Lermontov arrived at the hospital in his eight-cylinder Mustang, which made a terrible noise and had no radio or air conditioning. During the cold winter storms that dumped lots of snow, or on hot summer days, I used to ask him rather concerned, if he was still coming or going from that same floating shell. "It's a comfortable yacht, Sir!" he'd answer.

He lived there throughout the residency, four years in all, and during his vacations he would head back north towards Albany, where he had a little piece of land on a remote riverbank in total wilderness. With his own hands he'd built a little bungalow without running water or electricity. When he came back from vacations, his hands were even wider and full of callouses, just like a lumber jack's. There were no hospital gloves big enough to fit his hands, so they had to order special, oversized, gloves. On those boxes was written "Lermontov."

At the beginning, I was a little intimidated by him, but then I began to value and respect him because he did his job well, without complaints, or bowed head. At the end of the first year, which in fact he was repeating for the third time, he could perform a caesarean section by himself and administer the perfect dose of Heparin. At the beginning he called me "Sir," even though he was older and had blue blood running through his veins.

During a night shift while we were closing a woman's abdomen, I asked him if he'd ever been to Russia. He looked at me as if I were a mad man, because he'd never left the northern parts of New York State, nor did he wish to. After he started feeling comfortable working with me, he invited me on his boat. I returned from our trip with a big knot in my throat. We sailed out in the open ocean, far from the shore, far from our hospital, far from everything. Only then did his face brighten. He made a gesture at the boundless ocean in front of us, and all of a sudden he became a different man, looking taller, stronger, with another kind of expression on his face:

"If we're ever kicked out or get sick of all this hospital work we can run away, take to the world and live free on the land, on the water, or in a distant forest. Have you ever thought of that?"

No, I hadn't thought of that, although once in my youth I'd been lured by the oceans and forests. In the last years I'd fought so hard to be incarcerated by the walls of an America hospital that I could not see myself wandering free all over the world, other than taking vacations. Maybe I wasn't the free man I thought I was. Then I realized that Lermontov possessed some secret of life, which I, still too uptight in everything I did, have not yet discovered.

He kept an old framed sepia photo of his grandfather in a white tsarist uniform posing in front of a grandiose country manor in old Russia. I told him that many immigrants from Romania were going back after years and generations to reclaim old confiscated properties, which now are worth millions. He just shrugged his big shoulders, uninterested. Once he asked if I reclaimed some of my old country estates, and I told him that there was no such thing in my family, except for a few memories.

Lermontov often spoke Russian in the hospital because there were many Russians around. Shifrin and other native Russians were rather amused and recognized that Lermontov's language, although it sounded impeccable, was an old one, archaic, taken out of history's mothballs. Sometimes when I would bump into a Russian patient or someone from Bukhara, I would ask Lermontov to translate. When he spoke, the faces of those Russians would undergo a strange change, as if they were seeing an old movie or talking to a character in one of Dostoyevsky's books.

At that time, I was Chief Resident and we made some polite fun of America, my new country, where an emigrant like me could supervise and give orders to a noble man like him.

"Sir, God bless America," he said. "Perhaps you had to come here to be Chief."

One winter morning when we were putting on our scrubs in the locker room, a pistol fell from the back pack he carried every day. He quickly put it away and said that he and his wife never left their boat unarmed. They'd been robbed a few times on their remote property by local Catskill bandits, who were growing marijuana that he destroyed each summer when he got there.

One day the Chairman called me in and asked if I was aware that Lermontov brought guns to work. I said that I knew nothing about that but told Lermontov to keep his freaking gun at home until his Residency was over.

"A pistol can be more dangerous to your future than a wrong dose of Heparin," I told him bluntly.

When he finished his Residency, he already had a contract somewhere in Alaska. Alaska?! I knew that's where there lived mostly men, moose and bears. He shook my hand when we parted and assured me that there were enough women in Alaska for him, besides the forests and wilderness that he so loved. He said that from Alaska he might venture to Russia on his boat, even he was a little bit scared to go there. Russia was still a wild dangerous reality etched into his genes by the memories of his ancestors.

I never saw him again and know nothing of him, as I know nothing of the tens or hundreds of Residents who went through Jamaica Hospital, passing like fragile boats with their sails always pointed into the wind, ready to disappear in the unbounded hungry belly of America.

IT CAN'T BE!

FOR AS LONG AS I LIVED in Romania, I was afraid of uniforms because etched on them were signs of fear. Policemen wearing the low ranking uniforms could stop you in the street, ask for an ID, curse or even kick you for no particular reason, while officers in higher rank uniforms could harass you more perversely, like search through the files of your life as they pleased, files full of information completely unknown to you.

I was surprised when the Comrade Major entered the emergency room dressed in his military parade uniform. Having done my time in the army and myself being dressed in a white hospital uniform with a cap on, I instinctively gave him a military salute. He smiled almost paternally, and said jokingly, but firmly: "Loosen up, doctor! I brought my wife in who is expecting. Her water just broke, and I believe it's going to be a boy. We've been waiting for years."

Mrs. Major was about forty, a bit plump as many pregnant women are, dressed in a wide skirt that hid her protruding belly. She had all the stuff needed for her hospital stay: slippers, pajamas, a bathrobe, even a few sets of baby clothes which touched me. Those were the days when the sex of the baby was unknown; there were no ultrasounds, no genetic tests, and birth itself was still considered a dangerous adventure for mother and baby. According to our superstitions, it wasn't OK to buy baby clothes until the baby was born. A celebration like a baby shower was inconceivable.

I had a moment of hesitation because I was expecting that immediately after Comrade Major appeared, one of my bosses would show up, as the order called for. I was very young, recently arrived from my specialty training, and I knew that for the time being I had to stay put and be thankful to handle the wives of the lower ranking officers and the gypsy women from Garcin, a Gypsy ghetto close to the city.

It had taken time, obedience and hard work to get in the position to treat the wives, daughters or lovers of the more important people, because that could help establish good connections and could propel you up in the hierarchy early. At that time the most important patients were those who worked in the gas stations, grocery stores and even the sales women in the book stores. The economic crisis was getting deeper, with big shortages of food, gas, culture and freedom. The ones who cared more about minds and souls had retreated to the blurry world of books and self-education which were our only decent escapes, preferable to alcohol and madness.

I had no idea that Comrade Major was working in the passport section of the local police department.

"Doctor, I'm ready," said Mrs. Major cheerfully, already getting undressed behind a curtain. She was a pretty woman, freshly coiffured, with a youngish face, but heavily made up.

"Did somebody take care of you during pregnancy, madam?" I timidly tested the waters.

"No doctor," the Comrade Major responded for her. "My wife is a sensitive woman and is afraid of doctors. I didn't want her to get too traumatized before the birth... we suffered enough already!"

This was nothing new for me. More than half of the women who came to give birth didn't have any prenatal care. This happened during the mid-eighties when we hadn't yet seen an ultrasound machine or a pregnancy test, as we have today. Pregnancy tests were only done in the hospital and only using bullfrogs. The test, now history, was called Galli-Mainini, and the poor bullfrogs were already exhausted after so many tests performed on them. I could hear them during my night calls croaking sadly in the hospital's lab. Abortions were strictly forbidden, and women would hide unwanted pregnancies and have illegal abortions, trying to stay away from hospitals, doctors, and our bullfrogs, who could legally prove that they were pregnant.

During those days, we, the doctors, were afraid of uniforms like never before. That day I had in front of me a couple who wished very much to have a baby after having gone through lots of fertility treatments. I was scared and heartened at the same time. Before I could sort out my feelings, Mrs. Major jumped joyfully onto the examination table. I put my gloves on and gathered myself to examine her. As I was checking her, my face must have gone through a number of weird expressions, one more bizarre than the other, changes that didn't escape Comrade Major.

"Doctor, is everything alright?" he asked me nervously.

"Madam, when did you have your last menstrual cycle?" I asked.

"Exactly nine months ago. I wrote down everything in my notebook." She continued: After four months the baby began to move, my belly grew nicely, and this morning my water broke."

"Please relax your abdomen. Let me try one more time."

I reexamined her to make sure that I was not dreaming. Not a single sign of a pregnant uterus at term, an immense organ that couldn't have escaped attention. The relaxed abdomen of the lady was distended and large, but not because of a pregnant uterus. Her uterus was small like a lemon, the size of a normal and un-pregnant one. I slowly took off my gloves keeping my back towards them, thinking of how I should tell them the truth. I'd read about such cases, but this was the first time that I'd encountered one. Trying to avoid looking into their eyes, I spoke simply and chose my words carefully:

"I am very sorry, but I don't think that you're pregnant!" The words came out heavy, like dropping stones.

"It can't be," responded Comrade Major in a mix of utter confusion and anger. "What are you talking about? We came here to give birth, and you're saying that she won't? That's a good one! Don't you understand that her water broke? I want an experienced doctor! Who's the Chief here?"

"Doctor Fodor. If you want me to, I'll call him."

"Absolutely!"

I walked out on tip toes while the lady was getting dressed with big tears in her eyes. I was truly sorry for both of them, and I wished I could've made a miracle happen on the spot to resolve the biological confusion she'd lived through for nine months.

When the harsh truth or bad news comes out, it's usually the men who react badly. Women take it all a lot easier, but it's amazing how women sometimes may fully ignore the very signals that come from inside their bodies. Or how they can misinterpret them.

Women who wait a long time for a baby who doesn't arrive, can suddenly enter into a false state of pregnancy that takes over their entire being. The body keeps up with the subconscious and dutifully mimics pregnancy with all the transformations a woman goes through during nine month's time. They get sick and throw up in the first three months, feel the baby moving, which is nothing more but intestinal gas, eat twice as much, get a big belly, and as we've seen, their water even breaks, which in fact is a sudden loss of urine. Today it's hard to fathom cases of "psychological" pregnancies due to handy pregnancy tests and ultrasounds which put a halt to their wishful thinking before the nine months are over.

By the time I came back with my boss, the couple had already departed. I was left with a strange taste in my mouth and regretted that they hadn't even given me a chance to explain a bit more.

A few years passed by, and in the meantime, I decided to leave the country, to defect from my old life. At first, I tried to travel to Yugoslavia's Dalmatian coast and signed up for an organized tour to Dubrovnik. I knew that from there one could make it by boat to Italy. I waited for a passport for a few months, but nobody paid attention to me. At that time very few people were allowed to travel abroad. Three weeks before the possible departure date, I asked for a meeting with the local police at the passport office. To my surprise, the request was quickly granted. In the last few years there, I had managed to treat a few policemen's wives.

I dressed up in a suit and tie, and there I was, standing in a cold and forbidding waiting room at the police station. When you see so many blue uniforms all around, you become even more allergic to them. You haven't done anything bad, but a stupid feeling that you're automatically guilty becomes amplified in your mind. That's why, I believe, they make you wait so long. After an hour, I was called in, and I was face to face with Comrade Major who, in the meantime, had moved up in the ranks. He was absently thumbing through my file without looking at me.

"Doctor, take a seat. Tell me how many babies have you brought into this world? Is the birthrate growing in our county?"

Smiling, without a word, I gestured that what he'd said was true. He didn't like it.

"So, you want a passport to travel to the Dalmatian Coast?"

I confirmed by nodding my head. I couldn't find words. Meanwhile he lit a cigarette and inhaled deeply, looking at me over his glasses.

"Why do you want to travel so far? Isn't our seaside just as good? Yeah, yeah, I got it. You want to see something else. It's normal. But why the Dalmatian Coast?"

"I don't know" I shrugged, as if I made the decision by tossing a coin.

"Why not go to the Soviet Union? Sochi or Odessa? The Russians have a splendid seaside. I was there. Don't you think so? Maybe Central Asia: Tashkent, Bukhara, Samarkand. How about Leningrad and Moscow? It's a great country, very diverse. Any time you want, once a year!" Comrade Major seemed to be a tourist guide with the disposition of a comedian.

"I'll think about it. Thank you!" I got up and walked to the door. Just before I left, the Major turned to me, smiling: "Doctor, I forgot to tell you that we have a two-year-old daughter. It's true that we had to go to England to make it happen. It's a cold and austere country, believe me. But they do have good doctors. For us, here, you're pretty good, and we don't want to lose you."

I felt so "flattered," that I had to stay there for another five years. I do not regret it because at that time I had no clue about what it meant to leave your past behind carrying a suitcase full of mixed memories. All my attempts to defect were blocked. When I wanted to run away the Revolution came upon us. I got a passport and I was finally a free man.

BREAKING OF THE WATERS

THE BREAKING OF THE WATERS might be a sign of waking up to reality. The term "breaking of water" may be somewhat confusing, but very often we ask pregnant women if their water broke, meaning the amniotic membranes that separate the fetus from the rest of the world inside the uterus. When the membranes break, water pours out. From that moment, we know that the unborn baby will soon be born.

I didn't see many "psychological" or imaginary pregnancies in the U.S., but I did see many women who found out that they were pregnant only when their time had come, right before giving birth. The situations have been so many and diverse that they alone wouldn't fit in one chapter. It seems hard to believe that a woman who had given birth to five other children would find out that she's pregnant only minutes before she gives birth. But recently, this happened during one of my 'on-calls.'

The emergency service announced that the firefighter's ambulance, maybe the fastest and best organized of all the ambulances in the world, was bringing in a woman who was bleeding and who 'could be pregnant and even about the give birth…' That was confusing from the beginning. Was she or wasn't she pregnant? Even if she wasn't about to give birth, one thing was sure, she was bleeding, so we got ready for the task, our adrenaline increasing and getting instruments prepared in the Operating Room.

The storming-in of the firefighters through the hospital's corridors looked nothing short of an invasion, or rather a hastily organized retreat. The stretcher the woman was brought in on was almost broken, and she was being carried more on the firefighters' shoulders than on wheels. The patient had been tied to the stretcher with ropes because she was so obese that her body fat was hanging over the sides of the stretcher and moving in waves.

You can easily identify the legs, knees, neck or elbows of any patient placed on a stretcher, but when people get so big that body parts disappear in the folds of their own fat, any human shape and anatomical details may become almost unrecognizable. Although young, some women can get so obese that they have great difficulty leaving their beds or moving about the house. But amazingly they can still get pregnant, somehow defying the laws of biology or even the laws of gravity. There are a few parts of our body that regardless of how much fat we put on, do not hold fat: around the brain, the vagina, and the penis. At some point, this may save our species, considering that obesity in the United States has become one of our greatest public health threats.

Terrified, I looked at the fire fighters' entry, because I knew that these men must have had a good reason to have brought the woman to the Delivery Room.

No matter how it happened, delivering the baby of a woman of such proportions could become a serious and dangerous adventure. In the beginning, nobody asked how it was technically possible that a woman so big could get pregnant. We are professionals, and even when the danger is gone, we don't usually ask ourselves useless and mysterious questions. In the U.S., I've seen many enormous women get pregnant, seemingly by natural means.

Morbid obesity, as we call it today, may be associated with hormonal and metabolic malfunctions, leading to infertility, but women's fertility is something suspended in between science, magic, and the supernatural. For these women to gain another 45-65 pounds is but a tiny detail that goes unnoticed, and after delivery, no one may notice that something in their shape has diminished.

The woman was brought in by the firefighter's ambulance, which was the first one to respond. The firefighters were all tall, strong, massively built, as New York firefighters are, determined to see their mission completed to the end. They all looked scared, but seemingly unimpressed by the woman's dimensions or the idea of procreation itself. Later, she told us that half an hour before she was brought to us, the woman was in her house washing children's clothes in the sink when she felt something warm and wet pouring down from between her legs, feeling like a veritable thermal spring. She stood there perplexed for a few minutes until she began to feel pain along with the water which continued to flow and turned first to pink and then red. The firefighters arrived in five minutes, and one of them said from the start: "You might be pregnant, ma'am!"

"It can't be! It can't be!" she kept repeating. After all, she had five kids and she knew darn well what a pregnancy felt like.

It's quite difficult to examine these women because they can't easily get on the consultation table, and they have problems spreading their legs. The very thought of procreation might be hard to grasp. Not to the woman whom the firefighters brought in! She was close to five hundred pounds, but with the help of his brave colleagues, one of them, who had some obstetrical training, had been able to examine her at home. "Doc, the baby has a large head, but there is something else in there..." He told me as they lifted the patient onto our table.

For as long as the firefighters have brought us emergencies, I've never seen them screw up a diagnosis. They are straight forward men who would rather say nothing if they don't know. They all seemed ravaged by their experience with that woman. After all, they were well trained professionals, but men who'd rather deal with fires than women whose water broke.

The five men turned themselves into a human crane as they hoisted the woman up to the gurney. I examined her with great difficulty and felt the baby's head coming out, with one of its hands in the way, which complicated the whole situation. I tried to push the hand back into the uterus, but there wasn't enough space. I pushed back the baby's head; then I pinched the stuck hand quite hard. This trick works sometimes. Even if he isn't yet born, the baby feels the pain, and when his hand is pinched, he instinctively pulls it back. Not this time. I didn't yet know whether the baby was dead or alive, or whether he was already suffering because a suffering baby doesn't react. It was impossible to place a monitor on the mother's huge belly who, just like us, was completely taken by surprise about what was happening. She was quite troubled and couldn't believe she was giving birth.

I had to explain to her in a few firm words that the firefighters were damn right: she was full-term and a large baby was struggling to get out. She understood that very quickly. I told the Chief Resident, who was a short man of Asian origin, to put on gloves while I got myself together with a few other students, plus the firefighters, to try to keep her in the position that was needed for giving birth. She was so big that it took three of us to move one leg. Even her knees disappeared in the mass of fat, leaving dimples where they once were.

"C'mon mommy, push hard, bear down," we all screamed at her.

At some scary point the Chief Resident disappeared entirely between her legs like a man swallowed by fate. The woman took a deep breath and then pushed so hard that we were all thrown against the wall while the Chief Resident almost fell to the floor, holding the baby in his arms like a football player. The hydraulic bed the patient was on broke apart with a loud noise, leaving us all perplexed, drenched in sweat, amniotic fluid and blood, surrounded by a strange silence, pierced only by the screams of the baby.

The whole thing lasted four or five minutes. The neonatology nurses, scared as hell, tried to take the baby before the umbilical cord was cut, which had gotten stretched like a rope ready to be pulled in. I walked out to wash myself off. The firefighters were catching their breath next to a wall splashed with blood. I left the Chief Resident alone and he disappeared again between the woman's legs, trying to remove the placenta. Ten minutes later they called me back because the placenta came out intact, the uterus was nicely contracted, but the woman was bleeding heavily. I felt like running after the firefighters to bring them back, but it was too late. Although troubled by the event, they'd grabbed their gear and had rapidly disappeared, as if they'd been called for another emergency. The woman had to be taken to surgery to have a vaginal rupture repaired as soon as possible. I gathered all the available men I could find. I asked the anesthesiologist to put her to sleep, and we carried her as best we could to one of the Operating Rooms that had a hydraulic table especially made for heavy women.

After I managed to stop her bleeding, we all needed some time to re-group. Later, in the Recovery Room, after she came out of shock, the woman confirmed that she hadn't had the slightest hint that she was pregnant.

Her surprise, and ours, was not going to end just like that. After midnight other firefighters showed up—the night shift—carrying one of the woman's daughters. The daughter got so utterly scared by what had happened to her mom that she started to have intense stomach and head pains. She called the ambulance, and the same one came, which brought her immediately to the E.R. As the routine goes, they did lots of tests on her, and in the end the truth came out. She was also pregnant.

The same Resident called me terrified and gave me the news. I asked him to repeat it a few times to make sure that I understood. The Chinese have a special pronunciation, which lacks the consonants at the end of their words, making it easy to misunderstand them or not understand them at all. The truth is that immigrants like us complain more about others' accents, rolling their eyes more often than Americans do. I immensely admire the "locals" for their tolerance, and sometimes feel for them, because they hear their own language being butchered in so many ways.

I had an American colleague who came from Alabama, and who, before she got used to Yankee slang, was utterly confused by Russians, Chinese, and Indians whom she had to deal with. She learned rather quickly how to understand our words, and later on, even how to imitate our accents! At every Christmas party we would ask her to amuse us with her international potpourri of impersonations, where we could all recognize ourselves.

I didn't like it, but I understood what the Chinese Resident was saying. He had already done an ultrasound on the girl, and, surprise! In the girl's uterus was a thirty-seven-week old baby. The girl, like her mother, had no clue that she was pregnant and couldn't grasp the idea that there was another life in her womb.

Clearly they were both eating from the same food in the same fridge, because she was almost as big as her mom.

The results of the anti-obesity campaign in the U.S.A. are obviously far from having visible effects. Seventeen years ago when I started to work in one of the clinics, in the first month I had amassed a couple of complaints from patients. The boss called me in and showed them to me: turns out I had told a few patients that they suffered from obesity, which they didn't like. During those days the politically correct term was "overweight."

I examined the girl with great difficulty. She was already in labor and her cervix was dilated three centimeters. When I told her that she was going to give birth, she reacted just like her mother: "It can't be!"

In the end, she couldn't deliver vaginally because her baby was in a bad position, incompatible with natural birth. When I explained to her that she needed a caesarean section, she didn't understand a thing, but signed the consent form. Through sheer miracle, the baby's father showed up, a boy of about sixteen years old, with dropping jeans, baseball cap turned backwards, with lots of body tattoos, likely to increase even more in number after such an event. When he found out that he was going to be a daddy, he started to jump up and down with joy and called his Brooklyn buddies on his mobile phone, repeating:

"Guys, I'm goanna be a daddy! I'm going to be a daddy."

Because I had to explain in their terms what a caesarean section was, the baby's heart rate went down and we had to rush the mother to the O.R. The anesthesiologist quickly put her to sleep, and in no time I pulled out a nine-pound baby who screamed like any new born who had been taken by surprise. After she spent a few hours in the recovery room, I moved her to the same room where her mom was. The next day when I passed by, I noticed that the girl completely ignored the presence of her new baby who'd been brought in for nursing. She behaved as if she couldn't understand what relationship she had to the little being who was wrapped right there in diapers. She didn't even try to take a look at the small creature.

The Resident who was doing rounds that morning considered such behavior inappropriate and called the psychiatrist who called me shortly after.

"Doctor, the girl has no psychiatric issues," he said. "I hope you realize that she's only thirteen. She didn't have a clue that she was pregnant, or that while she was asleep you took a baby out of her. It will take some time before she'll understand what's happened. You should have called me to evaluate her mother."

The next day I walked into their room to check up on them. It was a nice quiet family scene. There was the grandma breastfeeding both babies, while the girl sat with a doll in her arms and was coloring a cartoon book, using markers brought from the Pediatrics section.

ARMY AND ABORTIONS

I KNEW WE HAD NO ESCAPE, and in the end we had to serve our motherland. Nobody got out of being drafted into the army in Romania, not even the doctors. I still have a group photo from back then, where it's hard to recognize me! A challenge even for my own parents! The uniforms, the caskets, the somber looks, the standing in stiff formation, made us unrecognizable.

As doctors, we had to serve for only four months. Nobody knew for sure what we were supposed to learn there besides marching in step, the military salute, and how to get used to a goofy form of discipline few people believed in anymore. The generations that followed suffered even worse. If they got into medical school, they had to do nine months of heavy army duty before they started their studies—everyone was drafted, with no exception, including young women, regardless if they were sick, or were pregnant. The unnatural selection began early.

The boys who did not manage to get into college right after finishing high school lost the chance to join the line of brilliant intellectuals with a diploma. At the age of eighteen, they were immediately drafted for nearly a year and a half. They would end up getting a few bad tattoos while in a drunk and existential confusion from which it was hard to escape. The factories and the agricultural fields of our motherland would greedily swallow them as soon as they were released from duty. The days when the army made you a man were long gone. What fantastic intuition my father had in those last days of December 1953 when he kept me hidden for two days only to register my birthday as being on January 1st of the following year to avoid me being drafted at eighteen.

Manu was my colleague in medical school, and we were in the military draft together. It was at the end of the '70s, and Manu reported to the military base in Bacau with long hair and a foot-long beard. I saw him entering the military base proud like a beatnik. He had round sunglasses, bellbottom pants, and a T-shirt that said "All You Need is Love." He looked like John Lennon on the cover of *Abby Road.*

He was grabbed right away by the military police and pulled into a cell as if he were a dangerous spy. Poor Manu was just another eccentric, an innocent civilian who only tried to imitate the rotten capitalists against whom the Romanian Army was supposed to defend the great Communist conquests from, although nobody knew exactly where the dangers hid.

When Manu came out of the barracks, he looked like a completely different man: in uniform, shaved head, no beard, without the round glasses, or the T-shirt that had on its back "Make Love, Not Children."

"What do you mean 'make love' a well-educated sergeant had screamed. "Do you think you came here for fucking?"

We quickly discovered that there were no women on the army base, and for the first time in our short existence we were going to go through a period when women were completely excluded from our lives. Many of us were already married and had little kids, and we'd already gotten used to what joy a woman could bring into a man's life.

During the first days of instruction, they would line us up in the morning and the Captain would cynically inspect our uniforms and haircuts that, by military code, were never in order. Either the mustaches or sideburns were too low, or the hair tucked under the beret was too long. After two days, we got fed up with that, and overnight, we gathered the whole platoon of misfit doctors into the communal bath where we cut our hair with a dull pair of scissors and then shaved each other's heads. The next day the Captain was furious, raging like a mad man. He knew that the army didn't have standard wigs in supply and whatever he'd try to do to us, he couldn't make our hair grow back right away.

"I'll make you curse the day you were born!" he said, then ordered us to run for an hour.

We already knew, from the previous batch of soldiers, that life in the army was not that dramatic. At least as long as we didn't overdo it. Our hair grew back slowly, as hair always does, and those four months in the army proved to be like a strange vacation in a bizarre camp. The best thing was that we didn't have to think at all, nor were our brains filled with anything important. A rare privilege that we wouldn't enjoy again in our lives! When we were done with fulfilling our military oath, an entirely different oath than the Hippocratic one, some of us were sorry that the draft had ended.

Manu slept in the bed right above mine, and I was glad that chance had placed me next to him because he was a quiet, educated guy. Plus, he didn't snore or play poker, or backgammon at night. We'd been colleagues before, while we were both in the Cluj medical school, and dorm mates for a while—that was until he met and married his wife, Dana, a colleague of ours, and moved with her to the family dormitories. They hooked up during the very first year when they were only nineteen years old. Having finally arrived in Cluj for medical school, we'd escaped the insufferable parental supervision, with our parents preaching only one lesson: stay abstinent until you grow up and get married.

Manu and Dana had been high school colleagues in the same Transylvanian city. Nobody and nothing could separate them. In the evenings, after they were done drilling anatomy facts from marked and torn books going back to the mid-forties, they met in the small park close to our campus. They could be seen behind a tree or on a dark spot passionately kissing and tearing off their clothes. The men from the veterinary dorm would scream from their windows "fuck her," but Manu and Dana couldn't care less. She got pregnant that year, and they were the first in our class to get married and have a baby who was cared for over the next five years by his parents.

During the first year, with all the school pressure, many colleagues hooked up just like Dana and Manu did, and the second year we had an epidemic of marriages among us. Because medical school lasts so long, some of these marriages fell apart by the fifth or sixth year when we were called to file for divorce. Manu and Dana stayed the same steady happy couple and made it together, after graduating from medical school, to their hometown, Arad, a city far away from Bacau, where the military base was located.

In our first month of duty we weren't allowed to leave the base or see any civilians, as civilians could compromise our minds with their shallow stupid freedom. Manu was the unhappiest guy. He kept a photo of Dana and his little girl in a pocket and looked at it sadly, as if we'd left for war.

"Calm down, man!" I would say. There are only twelve days left and our wives are coming to see us. Moreover, we heard that the married ones were allowed to go to town for half a day. In the end, the Romanian Army was quite reasonable and wouldn't tear the family apart, as they felt family was so useful to our sick society.

When the month came to an end, Dana showed up at the gate bringing Manu food, a bottle of good wine, and the room key to one of Bacau's downtown hotels. By six o'clock, the time we had to be back on the base, we were almost a full platoon lined up in front of the hotel, hastily dressed, happy and sad at the same time. Manu's eyes were tearful because Arad was a long way from Bacau and still there were three months to go. As for myself living closer to Bacau, I learned how to get a leave in exchange for a small bribe of a few packs of Kent cigarettes or a bottle of whiskey. The Army was not at all incorruptible.

Sometimes we wouldn't pay the bribe and would simply jump the military base's fence after evening classes where we were learning how to treat the type of wounds on people who'd survived a nuclear or chemical attack. We'd go to a semi-clandestine bar opened just for us in the backyard of a nearby house and have tripe soup and a beer.

The only one who never gathered the courage to jump the fence was Istvan, a Hungarian guy from the northern part of Romania, who'd sometimes behave rather weirdly, as if he didn't know us. He slept next to us, and when he spoke to us, he'd mix up our names, as he forgot who was who. Sometimes he used good Romanian; sometimes he spoke it awfully bad. We'd let him be because not all folks could adapt to the military life. Only after four or five years did I learn what really happened to Istvan.

One summer day I was walking on Mamaia's beach in civilian clothes when I bumped into a couple I knew well. That's when I found out that Istvan had a twin brother. They were both married and were both dentists and took turns doing their military service. Later, they immigrated to New York where they opened a dental office which they named "Twin Dental." I don't believe their patients ever knew who began and who finished their fillings. Anyhow, while in Bacau nobody could tell them apart.

After two or three months, I got used to the military. We'd play soccer in the evenings, smoke in the dorm which held eighty beds, where cases of beer would materialize, also look at porn that got there, God knows how. Pornography was forbidden because it was so damn imperialistic and could damage us physically and spiritually. That being said, the pictures were passed all over the dorm.

Starting at 5:00 a.m. sharp, we began our instruction because the most important thing in the army was to get up early and be kept in a useless alert state. The enemy was always at the gates, and, we, the active soldiers of the motherland, had to be vigilant. We did a few short target practices with AK-47s, a few interesting tactical maneuvers left from the First World War, and we took part in helping a flooded village near Bacau. We also strategically picked up apples and corn during the fall harvest. Overall, doctors were excused from services that required real guns and ammunition.

Manu had become rather absentminded and sad. He envied me because I left almost every Friday evening and came back Sunday from Brasov, where my two-year-old daughter was growing up nicely.

There came a time when our commander decided that we too could be used to guard the military base. The artillery engineers, who hated us because they served two months longer, six tough military service months, had to polish rusted cannons all day long—some old leftovers used once a year for a "secret" exercise at a well-known shooting range in nearby Fagaras. There, they would fire expired shells that didn't make it to Africa and Asia, places where our country was known to export lots of wheat, corn, guns and ammunition. The captain told us proudly that our country was well known for exporting arms. "Of the very best quality," he added.

At and around Brasov's mountain region there were lots of immense factories making tractors, trucks, mopeds, bicycles, batteries, sparkplugs and bearings. If one put those products together, one could also get tanks, cannons, Kalashnikovs, bullets, cannon shells and rockets. During my first days as a doctor in the Zarnesti Hospital, I witnessed something terrible. Rockets blew up in one of the local battery factories and the warehouse loaded with Katiusha rockets, ripping apart dozens of men who'd been sent to the hospital then home again in sealed coffins.

Shortly after my military service in Bacau, I was assigned to do gynecological checkups at Metrom, one of the factories that made bicycles, bazookas, and rocket launchers. Thousands of young women worked there. They were lined up and marched in, not necessarily for a real pap smear or gynecological exam, but mostly for detecting hidden pregnancies. We'd spectacularly passed the number of 20 million inhabitants, but since the seventies, Romanians had gotten stubborn and didn't want to multiply anymore. Ceausescu, who had banned abortions since 1966, was tightening the screws on the poor women who'd silently entered a kind of reproduction strike.

Most of the women brought for that strange gynecological exam were not pregnant. With the ones who happened to be, I would communicate through shared looks, but then I would write in the charts whatever I pleased. There were no tests for pregnancy, and they knew well why I'd been sent there. After a few visits they got used to me. I could examine a factory line of 50-60 women in only three hours. Their blue uniforms smelled of steel, gun powder and fear, but they didn't lose their sense of humor. When I'd walk in the waiting room, they'd shoot me hard looks and tough smiles. One of them would ask in a low voice "is he the one that's checking us for eggs as if we are hens?" Despite all this, I found lots of truly sick women, some with serious gynecological problems, who would later come as patients to the clinic where I was working. They almost all gave me the same present at the end of their consultation: a hunting knife with a handle made of elk horn. That was the under the table byproduct they made. "Doctor, it's the best quality steel," they'd assure me.

When we served in the army they summarily trained us to be guards, and the doctor's battalion was assigned to do night guard shifts at the military base.

"These are different types of 'on-calls,' little doctors! I hope this gets well into your heads!" screamed the captain. We each had an AK-47 with two fully loaded magazines. It was our turn to do the after midnight shift when we had to watch over a parking lot full of military vehicles. Manu and I were on the same shift, replacing the ones before us, by saying the military password, but only after they screamed at us: "stop or I'll shoot."

Manu ended up in a wooden tower at the opposite end of the parking lot. Under the light of the full moon, I could see him nervously pacing around like a lion in a cage. For the last few days he had been pretty grumpy, and I could hardly talk to him. It was a strange feeling to be alone in the night, isolated, with a machine gun full of bullets. We were two young men, armed to the teeth, against our wishes.

Our guns stank of steel, gun powder, and death! At least the wind, blown from the city, brought the fresh smell of grass and the scent of women. We'd sniffed them from the base like hunting dogs. For a few moments, I thought of my family. During those days I was smoking heavily. We weren't allowed to, but I lit a cigarette and puffed on it, keeping it hidden in my palm. The moon was casting strange shadows over the parking lot full of military trucks and jeeps, and I saw someone sneaking between them, getting close to where I was. There were still hours before I was to be replaced. I acted on reflex and screamed:

"Who's there? Stop or I'll shoot!"

"Stop shouting. It's me, Manu!"

I could see his face in the moon light. He had his hands in his pockets; his shoulders sagged, and he walked like a wet dog wandering the streets at night. He knew all too well that he wasn't supposed to leave his watch.

"I need a cigarette!" he said simply.

"Are you nuts? Where's your gun?" He motioned towards the wooden tower he had just left. I told him to go back right away, get his gun, and hold on to it, otherwise he might be sent to the disciplinary unit. He made a gesture telling me that he couldn't care less.

"What's wrong with you? What happened?" I asked him quietly.

"Dana is pregnant."

He looked so sad, as if something horrible had happened to her. I had never seen him so down and began to talk quietly.

"And what's wrong with that?" I asked him.

"Nothing's wrong with that! Only that she doesn't want this pregnancy."

"Let her get used to the idea. Wait until the baby starts to move. They all feel that way in the beginning."

He pondered a bit then said: "I don't know! I'd like to go home to talk to her."

I patted him on the shoulder, and after thinking a bit, I said: "We'll figure it out with the Captain."

I still had a few hidden packs of Kent cigarettes, and I gave Manu a cigarette that he lit from mine. When the ambers illuminated his face, I could see his scared eyes, his expression twisted by what looked to be dark thoughts.

"Don't worry, Manu! We'll baptize the baby next year. I'd like to be Godfather!"

Manu went back, recklessly holding the cigarette in his mouth, slowly dragging his tired feet.

I patrolled for a while because it had gotten cold; then I tried the door of one of the jeeps, and finding it open, I got inside to warm up. I played cool with Manu, but truth be told, we were constantly scared that our women would get pregnant at the wrong time. I placed the gun between my legs, I rested my arms on its nuzzle, and looking through the windshield at the full moon, I fell deeply asleep. During my whole time in the army, I slept better than ever, because during those non-medical night shifts, I knew that no woman would come to deliver in the military base. I had a long dream, a pretty civil one, a dream that would be banned by the army, if possible. In the dream, we were still students in Cluj. It was during the night when we all were studying for the tough summer exams, and all of a sudden, thousands of American Imperialists parachuted over our campus, which the whole city used to call Houston, probably because it had an old astrological observatory. In my dream, the Americans had surrounded the dorms and were summoning us to surrender because Houston was American territory and we had no business being there. We began to throw anatomy books at them, which we lit on fire, and they would explode when hitting the ground, spouting bones, viscera, nerves, and muscles into the air. Then our girlfriends came out from their dorm and began to scream at us to stop the bombardment because they'd willingly surrender to the Americans anyhow and would wave us good-bye as they left to send us postcards from the real Houston. The women were led by Dana, who was obviously pregnant and holding a white flag with blood stains on it.

I woke up abruptly when I felt somebody trying to take the gun from between my legs. Luckily its band got caught under my boot and I quickly realized where I was. I grabbed the AK-47, loaded it, and with my finger on the trigger, I screamed as loud as I could: "Move back, damn it, or I'll shoot!"

I jumped out of the car ready for battle. I had five guys in front of me spread on the ground on their bellies. "The password!" I screamed.

I couldn't remember what the password was, but they all said it at once, and then I stopped aiming at them and put the gun back on my shoulder. Then I shouted: "Sir, may I report: during my shift nothing unusual happened." I said it, as if falling asleep with a fully loaded AK-47 between my legs was something ordinary.

On the way back to the barracks they took my gun away and placed me in a jail cell. They took my belt, shoe strings, and all the other stuff that I surely wasn't eager to hang myself with. They confiscated the rest of my Kent cigarettes which I had intended to give to the captain in order to get some time off.

"So this is what you smoke while you are on duty! Doc, this time you've screwed up!"

Then, through the jail room window, I saw how the others were signing out, turning in their guns and ammunition. They would place the machine gun on the shelf, while repeating commands in a loud voice as if they were freshly minted Residents in an Operating Room. "Unload, pull the magazine out, no bullet left in the barrel, pull the trigger, all safe!" Then it was Manu's turn. Instead of doing it right, he shot a salvo of bullets into the sky. Knowingly or not, he'd forgotten to pull the magazine out. A bunch of different sized branches began to fall from the pine tree above. Scared, all the others threw themselves to the ground.

They brought Manu into the cell without his belt and shoestrings. He had a morbid look, and it wouldn't have surprised me if he'd hanged himself, if only he had the right stuff to do it. We stood there in silence all morning long. I couldn't get more than a few words out of him.

"Let it go, man, Manu! Things will sort themselves out somehow! If we get into the military jail at least we'll spend time in Bistrita where my parents live," I tried to joke. He continued to look at the ceiling. In front of the opened cell window fitted with bars where a soldier was patrolling was a kid of about 18 or 19 years old, a real soldier, one who was serving a 16-month term. I asked the soldier for a cigarette to share with Manu, but the kid played deaf. My cellmate, like any victim of extended torture who no longer reacted to pain, fell asleep with his face up. Two rows of falling tears joined at his chin, mixing with saliva and moistening the pillow stuffed under his head.

In our battalion there was a strange pharmacist who would read our fortune in whatever you wished: cards, coffee, beans, or our palms. "The future could be read in almost anything," he said.

Why not in some stains on a pillow," I thought.

The pharmacist had a guitar, and at night he'd play classical music or Beatles. Manu would constantly ask him to play "All You Need Is Love," and we'd accompany him obediently, "ra, ta, ta, ta, ta."

I slowly got up on the military cot inside the cell, and placing a finger on my lips, I asked the guard to approach but not make any noise. Manu seemed to have been taken far away to a future that was hard to predict. Ra,ta,ta,ta, ta!

I covered Manu with a blanket. The guard, who couldn't figure out what I was doing, got closer to the cell with an inquisitive face. I got my mouth and nose through the bars and using a foreign accent, uttered: "Fate, my friend is an old bitch, sentenced to an eternal life with its teeth lost, its fangs blunted, but ready to tear you apart." The soldier gave us a strange look, made the sign of the cross, then wobbled to a chair that stood in front of the cell, while looking straight at the blue linoleum, which we had to wash a few hours later. By midday they came and got Manu and woke him up from his sleep, slowly, almost gently, as if he were on Death Row and it was his scheduled day to die.

That was the last time I talked to him. In the evening they released me, and the sergeant, who was one of the doctors, told me to stay put because nothing would happen in the end.

"And Manu?"

"Same for him!"

I found out the next day what had happened because bad news travels fast. Dana, Manu's wife, had died in a hospital in Arad, due to an illegal abortion which turned septic and killed her in two days.

I remembered the day when we all went on leave to the hotel in downtown Bacau where we met our wives. That's when we noticed that all the Chinese condoms that could be found at any grocery store had disappeared. They were packaged in little boxes and had a tiny butterfly on top. When we bought them we would ask: "A Chinese butterfly, please!" The corner salesman would sometimes hand me one for change when I bought cigarettes. "They all flew away, dear soldiers! No more butterflies," we'd been told in Bacau that day. Condoms, the only contraception we had, were banned like any other contraception. That day we loved our wives with no protection.

When Manu left the military camp the lieutenant came to the dorm, picked up his luggage; then the guard at the gate called me to see Manu walk alone from the barracks. He was dressed in civilian clothes, wearing his fabled T-shirt and his round sunglasses. After a few steps he suddenly stopped and slowly turned his head. His face was spectral, bereft of blood and expression. He then began to wobble straight ahead. After a while his steps quickened and became steady. On the back of his T-shirt there was the same slogan: "Make Love, Not Children." I followed him with my eyes until there was nothing else left of him but a patch of T-shirt lost in the street crowd.

TERMINATED PREGNANCIES

IN 1990, WHEN I ARRIVED in New York, I used to walk the city for days. I wanted to see, smell, touch everything, because everything was brand new to me. I was like a house with all the doors wide open and all the windows broken by the winds of Communism's seclusion. I'd never seen a place with so many hospitals, one every few blocks, and private clinics in almost every large building. I thought that I'd come to a pretty sick world. It was soon clear to me that I didn't know everything about suffering, illness, and madness, in spite of the fact that I'd run away from a pretty sick and crazy world.

In the last twenty years, natural selection American style has thinned out the number of hospitals and clinics—a rather "unnatural" selection that the government tries to impose on the American health care system, an untamed-wild animal which slowly eats up our financial and moral resources. I believed that I was going to live in a country with a high quality medical system, but when I got here, I quickly understood that if you don't have some health care coverage, you're in trouble.

The competition is so intense in New York City that hospitals struggle to keep the patients they have and lure new ones from a neighboring area. With a little lack of foresight and mismanagement, any hospital may end up bankrupt because the people in that area have found out that they would be better served in a neighboring hospital, which might look like a five-star hotel, with a daily menu listing lobster soup, wireless Internet, cable channels, and many other little enticements.

Lots of hospitals have closed down recently. Those affiliated with the Catholic church were affected the most, while the Protestant and Jewish hospitals, better managed, have flourished. The empty buildings stay abandoned until they are demolished to make room for a new company, bank, or even a new hospital which may handle their finances more successfully.

When I came to America, I was surprised by the religious affiliations of many American hospitals. I came from a world where God was either forbidden, or kept on the sidelines, in the back room of a doubtful spirituality, perverted by fifty years of Communism. After its fall, God and Christ were brought out into the open with great fanfare by the very ones that kept them away. The people there are still waiting for the Romanian Orthodox Church, a wealthy and over-blessed institution, to build at least *one* hospital.

In 1992 I started working at Jamaica Hospital, a hospital that constantly grew, doing better and better every year. It wasn't and still isn't affiliated religiously or ethnically; in the chapel on the ground floor anybody can pray. A priest listens to confessions and may absolve any sinner. He holds a Sunday prayer that's broadcast on the hospital's TV station, and we have our "Jewish elevator" which on Shabbat stops on every floor because pressing an elevator button is forbidden for Orthodox Jews on the Sabbath. Across from the hospital there is one of the largest mosques in America; two blocks away is a synagogue and a large yeshiva for girls. On Jamaica Avenue there are a few different temples where on Sundays one can listen to gospel or a Santeria ceremony. But the most imposing building around remains the Queens Civil Court, which can be seen from the hospital windows like a landmark. We are praying to all Gods not to ever have to go there!

One of the reasons Jamaica Hospital is doing well is that it is often on the news due to unusual cases that end up in our Emergency Room, which is always busy. The neighborhood we serve is with no doubt one of the greatest human Babylons on Earth. Maybe that's why I never felt like moving to Manhattan or anywhere else. I like to travel, to see far-away places, with different people, different customs, but here, in Queens, we're all gathered in one single place. South Americans, Pakistanis, Russians, Chinese, Koreans, Afghanis, Poles, Romanians, Guyanese, Africans, Indonesians, each group with its tiny or large community, has its own quirks, idiosyncrasies and peculiar problems, which conspire to bring these people into our clinics and hospitals. It is an incredible human crowd that I never expected to mix with when I came from Europe. I intentionally say "Europe" when asked where I'm from. When I mention Romania, I get odd reactions. Some aren't able to locate Romania in their minds and mumble: "that's in Europe, isn't it?" "Yes, I am European," I would say with feigned pride. "I come from the world of white people, called "Caucasians" over here."

The Chairman of the hospital at that time, an Algerian Jew who was educated at the Sorbonne University in Paris, told me to be careful because being white and a man wouldn't help or put me into any minority group. "You belong to the "conquerors" he told me with irony, sizing me up from head to toe as I stood there, with no sword, no present, no glory, only some potential future hanging over my head like an illusion. Although he asked me very few questions, I was hired within five minutes. That's because I'd already been recommended by another Romanian doctor who worked at Jamaica Hospital. In the end, the Chairman told me one thing:

"Be careful with the women. Your colleague liked them too much and almost got himself into trouble. This isn't Paris, or your Budapest..."

"Bucharest, Sir!"

"Whatever, still Europe. I'll see you Monday at Labor and Delivery!"

Two years later, when I visited Germany for the first time, "meine liebe Europa," when I said that I was Romanian, I was skewered with cold looks, which would change when they found out that I was a New York doctor. America still had a good reputation in Europe.

When I see TV news vans around the hospital, I know that something unusual has happened. In those days, Giuliani, the Mayor of New York, had a little lectern with our hospital's name written on it, from where he would give TV press conferences, send greetings, or pass on condolences.

Two weeks after I started my Residency, I happened to be the one who handled a case that got plenty of publicity. For a whole week the newspapers had been filled with details related to a very strange abortion. When it comes to abortions, nowhere in the world does the topic spark more scandal and passion than here in the U.S.A. This delicate issue, overly abused in my own country, was one of the reasons that made me run away and cross the ocean.

I barely had gotten into the hospital system and was still trying to get the hang of it, mostly by observing what was happening around me. I was on probation, scared of the present, horrified by the future, and forgotten by the past, unsure of the English I spoke, my vocabulary still limited to the female anatomy. I was living from day to day, trying to reconsider many thoughts and concepts that I'd been avoiding to deal with for a while. It was a brutal form of conceptualization.

One night, the ambulance brought a girl who was bleeding into the E.R. She was eighteen and with her came her auntie, who, like the girl, didn't speak an iota of English. One of the big surprises I had when I started working in New York, was that I had to learn some Spanish too. In this case, I asked for a translator and found out that the girl had just "tried to have an abortion" in a private clinic in Queens. According to her story, the pregnancy should have been in the twenty-third or twenty-fourth week, meaning she was six months pregnant. I've never seen an abortion done at such an advanced stage. When the abortions were legalized in Romania, a pregnancy could not be terminated beyond three months.

I carefully examined the patient. Being at the very beginning of my American career, I had the strange feeling that maybe here in the States some other kind of natural order governed women's pregnancies. The girl's uterus was much larger than it should have been at twenty-three weeks, and through the dilated cervix, I felt something bone-hard and sharp, that almost scratched my fingers.

I took a deep breath, looked into the girl's eyes, and did something that I hadn't done since Romania: I bowed over and tightly pressed one of my ears to her belly because there were no old fashioned funnels around to listen to the fetal cord. I clearly could hear the baby's heart beating fast, too fast. I asked the girl again about her last menstruation and noticed that she was hesitating, asking her aunt something with her eyes.

I saw myself thrown back in time to my hospital in Romania where all the women coming in for abortions were hiding the truth. It wasn't even worth it to look for the truth because truth itself became a necessary secret. We were all hiding the truth. All we could do was try to help somehow, knowing that patients were never admitting how or when the abortion had been performed. Or who'd done it, what was used to make them bleed so badly, to get in such a septic state that brought them to the hospital almost dead. Eleven thousand women have perished during the twenty-five years when abortion and contraception were forbidden in Romania. Hundreds of thousands had been mutilated.

Back then, women feared doctors. They feared that we would document all details in their charts and would call on the authorities. I had chosen my profession because it was mostly about life, but towards the end of the eighties, it had become mostly about lies and death. We were working under the constant fear of police on our backs, just as now, in the States, our fear is of lawyers who hunt us down as easy prey. Back then, the police didn't "hunt us." They kept a vigilant eye over all aspects of procreation and would harass us only if we did something illegal.

What could that New York girl be afraid of? What was she hiding? Why did I immediately see fear in her yes and know that she wasn't telling the truth? After all, we were all now living in freedom!

Immediately, we took her to the delivery room where the Chief Resident did an ultrasound which showed, just as

I'd been suspecting, that she was carrying a baby of at least thirty-four weeks. It wasn't the first time a woman got to the delivery room not knowing how advanced her pregnancy was, or even if she was pregnant. The baby's heart was beating too fast, but then started beating too slow. We stopped asking questions because it was clear that both women were lying. One thing I didn't need to learn in America was to sense lies from a distance. I firmly told the girl that inside her womb was an eight-month old live baby who needed to be delivered immediately. The two women exchanged looks; then her aunt said that they'd just come from a private clinic where a doctor had tried to terminate the pregnancy. The very word hurt my ears! Terminate an eight-month baby?

The Chief Resident and I scrubbed in a hurry. That was one of the first caesareans I did in my new life in the States. My worst nightmare during those two years of interruption where I didn't work as an M.D., was that I'd forget how to do surgery. Some nights I dreamt that I got into an Operating Room and couldn't remember what to do. One of my colleagues, who went through similar anxieties, eased my fears, when he told me that surgical skills are like riding a bicycle. If you've got it, you'll never forget it. You may wobble a little at the beginning, but then you keep pedaling.

I'll never forget that caesarean section. The baby, an almost six-pound baby girl, was in transverse lie and was a difficult extraction. I barely could find one of the legs which I had to grab and pull out. In such a position, one of the biggest mistakes is to pull out one of the hands, because that would worsen the position. To be sure that you got a leg, you had to identify the heel by palpation. In that case, it would have been difficult to get a hand because one of them was missing.

It had been completely chopped off from the elbow down by the doctor who'd tried to terminate the pregnancy. The hand stub looked horrible and was bleeding. The girl survived and is still alive today.

It turned out that the eighteen-year-old mother didn't know that she was pregnant until she felt the baby moving. Her aunt took her to a gynecologist who did abortions up to twenty-four weeks of pregnancy. After they paid him a large sum of money, he rolled up his sleeves and started working.

That night I was completely exhausted when I left that 'on-call'. I took the subway where I saw the usual tired faces, bereft of any expression—mostly immigrants like myself heading to work in Manhattan like zombies. Their heads were moving like empty shells. I asked myself seriously: why am I here, what kind of world have I gotten into? When I got home I fell asleep, thinking that I should be patient and thankful to be back in a hospital and in an Operating Room. In a world that, in the end, should be better than the one I left.

That doctor who'd performed the late-term abortion was called "the butcher" and his name filled the newspapers and the TV news for days, stirring passionate ire in the 'pro-life' movement, who opposed any kind of abortion. One morning, hundreds of 'pro-life' demonstrators gathered in front of the hospital—well organized people, who were hysterically yelling slogans against abortion and the criminals who performed them. They carried symbolic coffins made for babies, grotesque dolls, pictures of abortions and banners that reminded me of the time when we, in Romania, were forced to march in demonstrations.

These people were not forced by anyone to get out into the streets. Their faces were contorted by fury and hatred, and I passed by, frightened, covering my work badge, so as not be identified as one of the "criminals." I remember the faces of two of the women, both around fifty, freshly coiffured, with heavy make-up, tight leggings and corpulent bodies. They were ranting at the top of their lungs, completely taken with their mission. I knew that from time to time a gynecologist who persisted in doing abortions would be murdered, or that abortion clinics had been bombed by such 'pro-life' fanatics. Ceausescu would have been their man, had they only known him.

One of my worst nightmares in Communist Romania was not only the lack of freedom, but the illegal abortions we had to face every day in the hospital. In the eighties the situation became unbearable. Most "abortionists" were people with no face, no identity, many with no medical training. Some women learned how to get rid of their pregnancies on their own, but most of the time, somebody else was involved. Once in a while, a dangerous, greedy, bastard came "on the market" like a serial killer, performing terrible abortions, leaving patients either in critical condition in our hospital, or having to be taken straight to the morgue. We were happy when we heard that the guy was caught by police. The news was not broadcasted at that time, rather it was spread fast by word of mouth.

Each time I'd been approached, and somebody tried to talk to me about "something," I had an inkling that it was about an unwanted pregnancy. I managed to convince a few couples to keep the pregnancy, and I delivered their babies. Most of the time, I wasn't successful though. I haven't done one single illegal abortion, and sometimes I did regret it. I think that I should have performed illegal abortions, just because some people close to me went through terrible abortions, done by untrained "professionals" on kitchen tables, or other dangerous situations. Money was not the issue. I earned enough practicing legal medicine, and then, there came a time when we couldn't even use the money we had because there wasn't much we could buy with it. We got closer to an immaterial world, one that would have produced glee in utopian socialists. Most women from my generation had an illegal abortion during their youthful years in Romania. To this day, I still listen to their horror stories.

On the very street I lived in Brasov, I had nice neighbors. It was a time when you knew the people who lived around you. Desperation brings people together, and that solidarity seems to have disappeared today in Romania. There was the pregnant wife of an Orthodox priest who lived three houses down from me. I saw her through her pregnancy, but I could not assist her at delivery because the Revolution happened unexpectedly and changed everything in the nick of time. As the shootings stopped in the streets, I got a passport, an American visa, and I was gone. I still look back at those days as a time of painful confusion. I bought a ticket, closed the door, got on a plane, and disappeared. How could I have done it so suddenly, I still ask myself.

Before I left, I knocked at my neighbor's door and told them that I wouldn't be around when she was going to give birth. It was a sad good-bye. The priest promised that he would pray for me, and I promised that I'd keep my fingers crossed for the baby to come out well.

There was one door, across the street, which I didn't knock on, even though I knew the people who lived there very well. They were a nice couple, both high school teachers, who had a daughter who'd just turned eighteen. I saw her growing up, playing in the street with other kids. Still an adolescent, she went to college, and then fell in love with a fellow student. One afternoon when I was walking in a quiet park, I saw them kissing on a secluded bench. They looked so charming, so deeply in love, lost in that magical world, the same everywhere, the one you rarely enter in life. Late in the evening he took her home and before parting got lost in a long kiss, right under my window.

I was then unsentimentally studying medicine until late into the nights in order to be sure I would be able to take and pass the American Boards when the time came. I had the feeling that the time would come soon. Had the Revolution not happened when it did, I would have defected somehow. I was ready to do anything, even cross the border illegally and dangerously.

When I was 'on-call' in the hospital I kept reading those medical books brought in from the United States. I kept the 'on-call' room door closed because I didn't want anybody to know that I wanted to leave the country, although I was on the "suspect" list. Almost all doctors were suspected, because our profession was recognized everywhere. Lots of my friends and colleagues defected somehow. Two interns from my hospital had been shot to death that very year, while trying to cross the border between Bulgaria and Turkey. That curbed my enthusiasm. While I was waiting for a false passport from my German friends, I was studying in the hospital. If somebody knocked at the door, I would hide the books under the mattress. Some believed that I was in there with one of the nurses, which nobody would report or consider abnormal.

One night I was called in the hospital's ER. There, on a stretcher, lay my neighbor's teenage daughter, unrecognizable, sick, pale, shivering with a high fever, her eyes deeply sunken. Her mother sat next to her holding her hand, slowly crying, sadly looking at the floor. No words were needed to understand what had happened. Somebody had performed an abortion by injecting chamomile tea mixed with vinegar into her uterus. Her mother quickly told me everything.

"We knew that you wouldn't do it! We found somebody, and this is what happened..."

The girl's abdomen was very painful and hard as wood. She had a septic abortion with generalized peritonitis, an easy and fast diagnosis. I went to the locker room where I had hidden a few doses of strong IV antibiotics and some special sutures, stolen from the military hospital. My hospital had run out of supplies. I knew that someday I'd need them. I tried to stabilize the girl and explained to both of them that without an immediate operation she'd die. They knew that. I also mentioned that I had to remove her uterus and possibly her ovaries. There were no questions. The girl agreed by nodding in resignation. No written consents were required, no explanations, no big notes in her charts.

Towards the morning I took her into the Operating Room. When I opened her abdomen, abundant smelly puss spurted out. I managed somehow to save one of her ovaries, which looked healthier. If she survived, that ovary would help her avoid menopause at eighteen. Most of the sutures I did not hold up well because the uterus and the surrounding tissue were dead. With a clenched jaw, I performed the surgery as quickly as I could, hoping that she wouldn't die on the table. I kept saying to myself: "oh, little girl, hold on, don't do this to me, now that I'm almost done."

Speed is important in these critical situations, because surgery itself is a big trauma and it may kill the patient. I removed her uterus and drained the whole abdominal cavity with improvised tubes, cut from some perfusion lines. We became the masters of improvisations. I washed her peritoneal cavity with all the sterile fluids I had at hand and left her vagina open for drainage.

How much unwanted experience did I accumulate in those few years, handling similar cases! How fast and precise was I moving that day, with a clock ticking in my ears! How absurd were my dreams of running away! All that I wished for that night was to see the girl stay alive. I felt like I was on a plane being shaken by strong turbulence at a high altitude when you're so scared that you feel like praying and promising to do all the right things in life, if only the threat ends.

The girl survived, but at what a price! I don't know what became of her over the years. I took care of her for the next two weeks. I pulled the tubes out of her body one by one, trimmed and dressed her infected wounds, and stole more antibiotics from the military hospital for her. Sometimes I just held her hand. It was hard to look her in the eye because I felt guilty. I don't know why. A few times I almost asked her: "why didn't you come to see me first?" but I kept quiet. What would I have done, had she come to me?

The Revolution arrived three weeks after the girl went home, and with it, the end of those times. The girl was skin and bones, a little bit hunched, and very quiet. She looked like she had aged twenty years. The day I wanted to say goodbye to my neighbors, I couldn't find the strength to knock on their door.

COMMUNISM, CAPITALISM, SEX AND LIBIDO

I GREW UP IN A WORLD where sexual problems were never discussed and sexual education did not exist in any form. In my youth, the only book about sexual education I saw was printed in 1938. During the whole span of Communism not a single book on this topic came out, as if sex and eroticism should exist sealed in our heads and reproduction was strictly a cerebral problem. Our leaders demanded as many children as possible and were betting against our primary instincts, which in spite of all deprivations, worked quite well.

Looking back from where I live now, I keep wondering how we grew up normal and, in the end, able to function in a world so utterly abnormal. It's even more mysterious to me why today there are so many dysfunctions amongst the youngsters in a world fully loaded with opportunities, education, and far fewer traumas.

In my youth there was no contraception or pornography: both were strictly forbidden. Videos hadn't been invented and for a kid, the only chance to see how a naked woman looked, was to go to a nudist beach in the summer, or later on, after we were grown up, to have a real lover who gave herself to you.

There was a bizarre radio program on sexual issues where both the questions and the answers were so veiled that one couldn't make much of it. Somebody explained to me that most of the carefully selected questions were referring to onanism, which was presented as some kind of underground subversive movement. Never called masturbation, an ugly word of capitalist origins, onanism (coming from Onan, a mythological-biblical figure) was harshly criticized by the materialistic-dialectic "sexologist," as being unhealthy and dangerous in all contexts. It was a veritable public enemy which could have derailed the normal evolution of Romanian kids and innocent young communists. Terrified, boys didn't listen to that program because it spooked and threatened them with all kinds of degenerative conditions of the spinal cord or other afflictions of the nervous system. "Be careful little boys, in Communism if you jerked off too often, you could become paralyzed!" I still wonder why they didn't declare masturbation illegal, like homosexuality.

As a boy, I wanted to initiate myself in the secrets of female genitalia. At least to see what it looked like. In my neighborhood, opinions varied amongst my friends. I had an uncle who was a dermatologist and found a colorful medical book in his library. I sneaked it out to study it with my buddies. It was a book about venereal diseases, and the pictures were so graphically gross that for a while we didn't want to know anything about sex and genitalia. One of us mentioned that in the summer, his parents used to bring him to the Techirghiol mud baths, where his mother would take him to a place where all the women were naked. He saw hundreds, thousands of them, but as they were covered in mud from head to toe, so details were skimpy.

The most read novel of Romanian literature must have been Rebreanu's *The Rebellion*, because we all knew that there was a scene, somehow erotically charged, when a landlady was caught by a rebellious peasant and raped in a furrowed field. The scene was pretty graphic for those days, and when I found the book in the school library, it opened to that particular page by itself. That was the extent of my sexual education.

Today, masturbation is not only not condemned anymore, but people with sexual problems are even encouraged by therapists to "explore themselves," in an attempt to pry open the Pandora's Box of sexuality. That box shouldn't be confused with the so called "Toy Box" that one of my American patients mentioned to me. She was an uninhibited woman who asked me if I would recommend a good vaginal lubricant she might use. She was a pharmacist and her question put me in a rather odd situation. I said that Johnson & Johnson's baby oil worked best as I learned from another patient, who laughed in my face when I recommended a product that was sold as lubricant. In medicine, a doctor may learn new things directly from his patients. My uncle, a Romanian dermatologist, had reached retirement age without having to trust any of the popular medical drugs, and he used to recommend cures learned from his own patients based on 'word of mouth' medicine and experience. My patient thanked me then and at the next visit secretly told me that she had added that oil to her "Toy Box." I didn't want to ask what else was in that box.

During my youth, sexual issues were taboo. The "Toy Box" of the Communist regime was dead empty, and whatever could be there had nothing to do with sexuality. Rumor had it that in schools, campuses, army barracks and wherever youths would gather and eat, the government put bromine in our food in order to keep our sexuality in check. I went to student camps, I lived in student dorms, I've been in the army barracks, I ate their food, but I didn't feel any effect from bromine.

It seems that today young folks are even more "bro-mine-ed," and I often ask myself why? Could it be stress, the new public enemy, all kinds of worries, plaguing us? Or is it due to the very exciting, but mostly virtual life the youngsters are immersing themselves in? These days, we're watching and observing life on a screen, pulled straight out of our pockets, and voila, the whole world is ours, an illusion we can control with our fingertips.

Even sex can be had on the Internet nowadays. One of my patients told me recently that she wants to get divorced because she caught her husband having sex with an Italian woman from Milano. In their own bedroom, over the Net. She had to explain a couple of times how it happened because I was more than puzzled. I felt completely overwhelmed by the whole story, like an old fashioned man stuck in a prehistoric romantic time. Sexuality during those olden days still kept its intimate mien and even its sacredness, which today is on the verge of being lost due to the ubiquity of sexual information readily available to any child who enters puberty.

Sex used to be nobody's territory. You could get there being carried by the tugging undercurrents drafting under the door of our natural instincts—that cracked door, only partly closed to leave just enough room for exploration. Once in that "no man's land," somehow we managed to find each other as we were, almost blind and disoriented. It was a zone with no words, no precise rules, the meeting place where we could declare peace to each other, or at least sign a temporary truce with life. We sniffed and touched each other discreetly, leaving traces in that fertile field where any seed could sprout to life. Slowly we learned how to walk, some tiptoeing, others trotting roughly with their boots. Sometimes we'd stick our flag of victory in the sand, or we'd just retreat into the surrounding world where we'd patiently wait for night to fall. The fall of the night, not darkness, not fog or those blinding lights full of symbols, stimulation, or sexual interdictions that could flood us. Today sex is no longer that hidden-magical territory. It's everybody's territory, a fenced alley full of traffic signs and directional signals.

There are still islands and isolated Asian communities in the Pacific where children begin their sexual life at twelve or thirteen. Parents encourage them and build the so called "love-nests," little huts on the edge of the village erected on bamboo stilts. The girls are the ones who lead this ancestral game of mating. As soon as they enter puberty, they are urged to choose a sexual partner among the boys who come and visit the huts. It's all done by instinct, combined with some parental advice. Of course some get pregnant, but the couple and their children are accepted by the whole community, even when it is not quite certain who the father is. There is no contraception, nor are there abortions. The girls nurse as long as they can because it's good for the baby and because nursing is the only natural contraception they know. On these islands the institution of marriage has not yet been invented, nor has divorce. The word 'jealousy' doesn't exist in their vocabulary, and people respect each other and love freely, with no official contracts. Old people complain that since the mobile phone came along with pornography, the old practices are not being kept by the younger generation.

Nowadays before reaching puberty, the kids have already seen porn on the Net and think they know all there is to know. Girls mature faster than boys and start their sex life earlier than parents can even imagine. Today parents talk openly to their children about sex in order to protect them. Protective and suspecting mothers bring their daughters to the gynecologist, but girls don't reveal much if parents are present for the consultation with the doctor. Sometimes they completely surprise me with their sexual confessions, and I try to protect them by offering a bit of sex education and advice, most of it already known. The old sex taboo has been completely abolished. As soon as zits appear on their faces, their schools, acting with foresight, offer free condoms, which the students carry as some bizarre talismans that would protect them against venereal diseases, all the ailments of the world, plus unwanted pregnancies.

In New York, I still see many 13 to15 year-old pregnant girls who come to the hospital's clinic for prenatal care during the school break along with the babies' fathers who are schoolmates. Some have two to three children by the time they are out of their teen years.

On the other hand, there are the old liberal Europeans, who have been completely taken in by an existential selfishness that moves democratically from Siberia and Scandinavia all the way south to the Mediterranean. Europeans don't want to reproduce anymore, even if every new census scares them to death. The reproduction strike began in my country long ago, but sexuality was always a welcome refuge. When sex was the topic, people spoke either trivially, or very delicately. People were still "making love." Now they have sex. Everything about it is well known and talked about.

The first notions of sexuality that I got rather involuntarily came from one of my colleagues during the '80s in Romania. Dr. Bota remains one of the most interesting people I've met in the first part of my life—a man who managed to escape from the monotonous and uniform atmosphere of that time. We worked together in the hospital and then in a strange clinic that I still dream of, as you dream about places that haunt you. During those days, sex and sexuality were fluid notions that you couldn't approach in the ways we do today.

Towards the end of the eighties something strange happened in our city. Although Communism had settled itself as an eternal and incurable disease and the medicine we were practicing fell behind the times due to shortages of all kinds, the authorities opened up an unexpected new type of clinic called a "Payment Clinic" where the patients had to pay a fee for our service. Overall, healthcare in Romania was free, covered by the government from birth to death, which were both officially granted to us. Only burials and the after-life didn't fall under the system's patronage. We became so "socialized" that nobody cared for us anymore.

The notion of official payment for services became a utopia even though many patients paid us under the table. Authorities called that a 'bribe' and declared it illegal. There were doctors who asked for money before a service was rendered, and one could go to jail for that—a parallel world, unofficially accepted, which continues its existence with even greater success today. Perhaps that's why the authorities came up with the idea of the "Payment Clinic," so they too could get their share. A consultation fee was 50 *lei*, the equivalent of 4 dollars nowadays, out of which we received a given percentage. The idea of such a "private" island in a world where private property had been almost abolished and free enterprise was considered a sin, seemed completely out of the norm.

The good thing about that clinic was not the money, but the goodies brought to us as gifts that were not considered bribes. Country women brought food: eggs, meat, cheese, which was much better than money because food was in very scarce supply in those days. The city ladies brought us Western cigarettes, coffee, whiskey, all somehow procured from the "duty free" shops even though only foreign citizens could make purchases there with hard currency while Romanians were not even allowed to possess any such currency. (For years I kept two hundred dollars hidden away, the only money I had when I came to the U.S.)

As expected, a question might arise: could sex exist in such a world? I can testify that it did, and abundantly so. Just because we were living in a society where there wasn't much to do, sex, although a dangerous adventure, became a veritable safety valve, often abused.

Towards the end of the '80s, the general feeling was that of an authentic end-of-the-world scenario. I'd read a book about the ancient Vikings who'd just been converted to Christianity. The missionaries drilled into their heads that the world would end in apocalypse around the year 1,000, and then they would all go straight to heaven. Nobody worked the land that year; they ate all their food, drank beer, and desperately loved their women. Most of the women got pregnant in the process of waiting for the end. About the same thing happened in my country during the last desperate days of Communism, only we thought that regime would last forever, even in the afterlife.

Working in that "Payment Clinic" I realized that people also had serious sexual dysfunctions. That clinic was subjected to all kinds of shortages. As was happening in the entire city, the electricity would go off during the winter time at about 6:00 p.m., just when darkness fell. At the clinic entrance, we were given some kerosene lamps, then we walked upstairs, where there were 10-15 extremely small consultation rooms. We continued down a long narrow corridor where patients were waiting, leaning against the walls, since there was no waiting room. Moving along the corridor I could see women's sunken faces, their shadows projected against the wall. They all looked like potential victims of crazy Manole the Mason-builder, who, according to our legend had to wall-in his own wife to make a monastery stand. All the walls Manole the Mason had raised during the day would crumble overnight, until an angel told him that a woman needed to be entombed alive, and she should be the first woman who showed up the next morning to bring food to her husband. These were the kinds of legends we were taught in school.

The "Payment Clinic" building was quite old, constructed at the end of the Nineteenth Century. In every room there was a tiny desk on which I would place a lamp, a narrow consultation table, a chair on which women would put their clothes, and a puny sink with only cold water. The room was cold, and women had to get undressed quickly, right in front of my eyes, since there were no curtains or gowns to cover their naked bodies. Intimacy or privacy, Latin words, in Romanian "*intim*" and "*privat,*" were just not part of our vocabulary any more. The rooms were connected to each other by small doors, which made the atmosphere even odder. There were no nurses to help us because there wasn't any room for another body to fit in. Still, it was the only place where women could come and see a doctor with no fear that they'd be spied on or recorded by others.

Dr. Bota, who was past retirement age, saw patients in the next room, which had "Sex Therapy" written on the door, and because of the thin partition between rooms, I could hear most of what was said there. I thought that those doors were there on purpose so that we could spy on each other. After all, that had become a way to keep things in check, a method that worked well for many years during Communism. People censored themselves and turned others in with great success, so there was no need to bother with microphones or other old fashion ways to eavesdrop. We became "wireless" long before it had been invented.

Across the street from our building was the military base for a mountaineering regiment which had stayed the same since the days of the Austro-Hungarian Empire. I still remember Dr. Bota walking in that dark clinic with a kerosene lamp in his hand. He looked like an old magician who didn't want to show all his tricks, a fakir who just came out from his bed of nails with an ironic smile on his face.

Many of the women who came to the clinic were pregnant, and most consultations were for pre-natal care, which was done by performing a manual examination and listening to the baby's heart beating through a funnel. Many women came there to test the waters for the possibility of having an abortion.

Dr. Bota came from an old family of Romanian intellectuals who traveled the world and were well educated before they got stuck and isolated in Communist Romania. His father lived in Vienna and had been to India to study Ayurvedic medicine, Hindu and Buddhist philosophy, and some Kama Sutra also. Dr. Bota had good ideas about all of these things, although they didn't fit in our hermetical world. In his house, the rooms had not been painted for decades because the walls were fully covered with books and paintings all the way up to the ceilings. He was one of those few people who not only succeeded in surviving and keeping his mind and wits intact, but also succeeded in diffusing light around him, giving the impression of an electric bulb that refuses to burn out. He was the first person who told me about yoga, meditation, and how important it is to breathe right.

When we were 'on-call' together, he would meditate in the lotus position and could do a head stand for a long time. His eyes were alive and expressive; his profile was as aquiline as an eagle's, and his hair was dyed black and pulled behind in a ponytail. Nobody had a ponytail at that time. He was married to a very young nurse from our hospital. They adored each other, and she took good care of her older husband. She became a stylish woman who dressed, talked, and behaved as if touched by an unseen world.

Dr. Bota was practicing something no one else had done in our city up to that point: sexology, and his small office was constantly busy. Because I could hear what was being discussed through the door, I became vaguely acquainted with what sexology meant, a specialty completely ignored in a country that wanted children regardless of how. When I asked Dr. Bota how he had come to learn sexology, he told me that besides his own experience, he did it by reading many books and foreign magazines. I had no clue how the books got to him.

"If they want babies, poor folks must get sex education, damn it! I convinced some people about this need, and I arranged that nobody would stop the magazines I get through the mail from the West. Along with the magazines, I also get some other books and articles that I'm interested in."

He spoke four languages and was very passionate about parapsychology and hypnosis, murky practices that escaped censorship and which were neither encouraged nor banned for the simple reason that they were beyond the feeble comprehension of the Communist Party, as was the case with jazz, which proliferated spectacularly in Romania's underground scene. Moreover, the hospital allowed him to practice hypnosis on some patients, and I saw him putting women into a deep trance a few times. Once he hypnotized an intern and made her sweat on only one half of her body.

In the clinic, surprisingly, most of Dr. Bota's patients were men. Silently waiting in the narrow and dark corridor of that clinic, they seemed to hide themselves, slipping even deeper into the walls. Some were waiting in the street for fear of not being seen there. It had never occurred to me that men might have even greater sexual problems than women. Their tough and rough lives, filled with brutality, sunk into alcohol, cigarettes, and domestic violence, had left a mark on those men's sexual lives. In our world, women seemed to have fewer sexual problems, and they mainly complained about men.

What I remember from the discussions heard through that door was that "men could not perform, and women couldn't feel." I don't know how in the end Dr. Bota dealt with all these problems, but there was always a long line at his door.

As a gynecologist, I often face the delicate situation of being asked to cross the thin line between gynecology and sexology. Sometimes, it's an awkward and uncomfortable crossing because I don't know what to expect on the other side or how far I'll have to explore.

Patients sometimes ask for my opinion when I least expect it, coming up with unusual details about their very intimate lives. Sometimes they just want to talk, to confess, other times they want to hear my opinion. After all, I am their gynecologist! I have no clear guidance about how much I should get involved in such issues, though I let common sense guide my judgment. American doctors receive some training in this field, but most of them seem to avoid the issues of sexuality. "Sex is in the head" most gynecologists would say, a place far from our specialty. After we reassure the woman that she has no physical problems, we are ready to send her to a sex therapist.

Before shifting to the electronic data system, clinics in New York had a questionnaire about gynecological issues that contained queries about the sexual practices of the patients. Among the questions were some like: "Are you sexually active?" "At what age did you start your sexual life?" "How many sexual partners have you had?" "Do you have pain during intercourse?" "When? In the beginning, during, or after?" "Do you have orgasms? Easily, with difficulty, or not at all?" "Have you been sexually abused?" etc. Ever since I was a Resident, I've thought it better to skip these delicate questions, and I believe I was right. It's one thing when a woman asks for advice related to her own sexual problems, but it's a totally different thing for a doctor to intrude in her privacy. Especially, if the doctor is a man.

I once asked one of my female American colleagues if she'd been using that questionnaire about a woman's sex life. She shrugged her shoulders and said that she only uses it when the patient asks for it. Sexuality may be a forbidden territory you never know what or whom you might bump into. Possibly you might even uncover admissions from that mysterious stranger that is always showing his back to us, the sub-consciousness.

She was still a very beautiful woman, even when she was about to give birth. The big belly didn't at all lessen her silhouette. She almost made you understand why some Hollywood stars dared to pose nude, even pregnant. There are many beautiful pregnant women, and if there were a beauty pageant for them,

I'd love to be a judge. My patient was originally from Slovakia, just over thirty years old and looked like a pregnant model. She always came to the office with her husband, a tall, elegant man, with the fine features of an Italian actor. Rarely did I see such a beautiful couple. They were clearly made for each other. Married in their own country, of which they spoke with great pride, they emigrated years earlier because they got the chance to work as architects for a large Manhattan firm. They seemed integrated and happy with all that they'd accomplished in the States, even though their faces had a vague trace of nostalgia and a smile that did not open too wide, not like the free smile of those born in the U.S. Anyhow, I didn't see very many immigrants with large smiles, at least not in their first years, even if they felt like they were in heaven. And if heaven does exist, I do believe that even there immigrants would need a long time to adapt.

When my Slovakian patient delivered her baby naturally, I must say that the painful and harsh process ended up being elegant and tender. Yes, a vaginal delivery may be like that, and regardless of how it is, it surely remains an uplifting experience, one that can move even an ageing obstetrician. It was a birth that I'll remember, even though nothing unusual happened, or perhaps that's the reason why I'll remember it. I asked the father to cut the baby's umbilical cord and congratulated and hugged them both; then I walked out of the Delivery Room with a good feeling, emotional, as when one walks out of the theater where the actors managed to bring you to a rare state of catharsis. Indeed, Delivery and Operating Rooms, with all their drama, blood, and sometimes violence, manage to bring us to such emotional states, at least compensating for the stress and exhaustion we go through when 'on-call'.

After six weeks, when I saw the couple in my office, she looked a little tired, with bags under her eyes and some emptiness in her look. I could see how the seeds of a mild depression had started to sprout. After they finally deliver, many women go through short bouts of depression, called "postpartum blues" that usually resolve themselves in time, without any treatment.

The brain of a woman has numerous receptors for estrogen and progesterone, hormones that during pregnancy increase hundreds of times. After the baby and placenta are delivered, all these hormones suddenly drop. It's actually a miracle how women succeed in maintaining their mental balance after going through such a huge hormonal fluctuation in such a short time.

A man's brain also has its receptors for masculine hormones, but our brain is subjected to a constant even flow, not being affected by some other cycle, such as menstruation. Not to mention pregnancy, birth, nursing or menopause. If men functioned hormonally as women do, we would probably witness a continuous emotional cataclysm that would threaten our species. Certainly there would be more divorces, crimes, wars, and sex itself might become an unpredictable adventure.

When I asked my patient what kind of contraception she would like to use, she looked surprised. She just said that she didn't need any. I asked her if she wanted a second baby soon. With a small grimace, she said simply:

"We don't need contraception, for as little sex as we have!"

I couldn't help but ask her:

"How often do you have sex?"

She took a long break, as if she was trying to count something, or solve a complicated puzzle.

"Rarely. Once, maybe two or three times a year. This pregnancy was like a miracle! I don't know... Since we got here, everything has changed. We barely touch each other. Otherwise we are perfectly fine, doctor!"

I was speechless. It was hard to believe and conceive that these two superb young people, beautiful both in body and soul, were not touching each other at all. The idea of being affectionate, not necessarily for sex, seemed to me to be fundamental in the relationship between a man and a woman, regardless of age.

She wasn't the first young patient of mine to come out with such an unexpected confession. Sometimes it was delivered with sadness and grief, sometimes with cynicism or a weird sense of humor. Each time I became rather disturbed, having had a strange feeling that we are on the edge of some kind of alienation that might be the beginning of a desert draught.

"Doctor, do you think *this* is unhealthy for us?" I heard the unsure voice of my patient, who didn't call "this" abstinence or lack of sex. I said nothing, because there was nothing to be said. I couldn't care less about all the political correctness and how a doctor ought to respond to such questions. Is it healthy or not to have sex?! I don't believe that was the question. For me, it just seemed terribly sad that these two young people got to the point of not desiring each other physically. It was a kind of involuntary sin against their own human nature. How could I convey such thoughts to my patient? Everybody knows statistics show that people who have a normal sexual life live longer and better lives. Then my patient added with a trace of guilt and relief in her voice:

"We got used to this and now it seems normal… Since we started working here, something has curbed our appetite… I don't know why; we lack nothing. Maybe stress, worries, the mortgage, bank credits? We get home late and are so tired…

Living back in Bratislava was tough; we had almost nothing, but it was different. Though doctor, contraception doesn't make sense to me…"

I had the feeling that she was sorry for the confession, and I said nothing else. Their situation was after all a happy one because they both shared the same abandonment of sexuality. Their libido had died equally for both, reaching an almost symmetrical asexual state, without suspicions, jealousies, or frustration. When their contract had ended and their work visa expired, they came to say good-bye. I believed they would go back to their country, but they moved to Canada where they'd been accepted unconditionally. I haven't heard from them since, but I'm sure they'll stay together because they loved each other, and love cannot be discounted in the equation of sexology. I still hope that by changing their environment, their physical relationship might have changed as well. Because of them and other similar couples, I started to pay more attention to the sexual problems of my patients.

MADELINE

UNTIL THE BABY STARTED to look like her, Madeline was never sure that the boy was hers. She would often wake up at night, turn the light on, and take long looks at him. What if the hospital had given her the wrong baby? The night he was born, five women delivered, and it wouldn't have been impossible to mix up the newborns.

When she was breastfeeding, he was too close to her eyes and heart, to truly see him. He would nurse for an hour, and during that time Madeline was completely transformed. She would keep her eyes shut and would think of nothing, her mind wandering to a strange no man's land. Her breasts grew nicely, and she liked when Bogdan, her baby boy, suckled them hard. Her husband was going crazy, and it was not easy to tell him that her breasts were no longer his. For six weeks she could avoid him because of her nursing; then Madeline simply asked him to sleep by himself in the living room. Her husband was a good man. He took good care of them, didn't drink, got up early in the morning and went to the factory where he built prefab walls that would be used to raise standard buildings all over the city—identical walls which would be placed on top of each other for many years to come.

She didn't tell him what had happened at the hospital the day she came back with Bogdan. To her husband, the most important thing was that he had a boy. That had been his wish.

After she gave birth, their relationship slowly began to fracture and would never be the same. Many women change physically after they have children, and their priorities change as well. The father might not be on top of the list anymore. Madeline transformed herself, becoming more of a woman who saw life through different eyes. The birth unleashed something in both her mind and soul. She rarely used to cry, but now would burst into tears for no reason. A good movie on TV could be enough, or even the sight of a bird who came to find food on their balcony. Sometimes she thought that she didn't understand much about her life, which up to then had been going in the direction she expected. Then, quietly, she cried. For a while, she felt as if behind her eyes she held a hidden lake keeping all the tears that had not been shed. She would look at Bogdan during the night, and although her doubts did not disappear, she was at peace with the idea that despite whatever could have happened at the hospital, as long as she was nursing and raising him, he was her baby and her baby only.

"Madeline, why do you stare at the boy?! It's like you are looking at the moon. I hope you won't cast a spell on him," her mother would say.

The day when they left the hospital, she had waited with other women to get their babies, all wrapped in diapers. It was cold outside, and the faces of the newborn babies were covered with a cloth. When Madeline got her baby, she grabbed him in a hurry and wanted to run away. Her mother, their guardian angel, was there as well, and wanting to kiss the baby, uncovered his face, but then said something terrible: "This is not our boy!"

Madeline was still dizzy after the morphine she received that morning, but her mother quickly took the baby off her hands and turned to the nurses who were checking the babies out and screamed loudly. "Where is our boy? We want our boy!"

The baby had an identification tag tied to his hand, but Madeline didn't have hers anymore. She'd torn it apart the night before when the wound hurt her just as bad as it had on the first night. Soon it came out that the boy belonged to a woman who still had her identification tag on her wrist. How guilty Madeline felt! She'd missed the birth of her own baby, so she couldn't see him right after delivery! She'd struggled a whole night with her labor pains but in the end she had to be taken into the Operating Room for an emergency caesarian section because Bogdan's heart was not beating well. The anesthesiologist quickly put her to sleep. When she woke up she was taken to the Recovery Room and kept dizzy and out of this world on morphine.

Madeline was only nineteen and her tolerance for pain was pretty low. It was hard to take any pain since she had had an abortion with no anesthesia—performed by a former nurse at home, right on the kitchen table where she'd laid herself out like a piece of meat ready to be hacked. She was seventeen and had gotten pregnant by her high school sweetheart, her first love. Her mother, her guardian angel, had convinced her to terminate that pregnancy.

"Madeline, Madeline, you don't need this baby now! You haven't finished high school. You are not even married, my girl."

After the abortion, or whatever that was, she could not enter a kitchen for a long time and could not return empty glass bottles to the store because they had to be cleaned inside with a special brush. Madeline was convinced that the nurse who'd terminated her pregnancy had used that kind of brush to clean her womb. Later she met her husband who was a construction engineer, a polite man, with no vices, who built nice identical prefab walls.

Once she had the caesarean, Madeline stayed in the Recovery Room for three days, with a fever and high blood pressure. When they moved her into the postpartum room with many postpartum women, she was completely exhausted. The women asked her how her delivery went, but she replied that she had no delivery because her baby was brought into this world by other people. She would point to the doctors and nurses. She only saw Bogdan three days later, and her mom took care of him. That day, they'd almost left the hospital with another baby, had her mother not caught the mistake.

"It's him, it's him, trust me," her mother kept saying with absolute authority. Madeline was still out from morphine and said nothing. They left the hospital in silence and hadn't spoken about it for years.

I was the one who delivered Madeline's baby, even though she kept saying that she'd never given birth, only that I took the infant out of her.

One day by chance I met her mother who complained that Madeline was getting weird. She would cry out of the blue, or stay silent and stare at the boy for a long time. She'd also neglect her husband, a nice man, and would write strange things in her diary. One day they found her on the balcony of the tenth floor looking into the void below. When her husband asked her what she was doing there, she said that she wanted to fly away one day once her wings grew long enough.

"What do you think about all this, doctor? We're all terrified! In the beginning she was obsessed that they'd switched her baby; now she wants to fly," her mother said. I told the mother that women in postpartum can enter forms of postpartum depression that could be mild, but also become very dramatic.

"She keeps saying that there's nothing wrong with her. I asked her to see a psychiatrist, but she refused. Could you please talk to her? She's gotten used to you."

I saw Madeline a few days later, three months after she'd given birth, or as she liked to put it "was delivered." In the States, at such time the discussion was mostly about contraception, but in Romania's '80s, contraception did not exist, even worse, it was forbidden, removed from the medical school curriculum, expunged from dictionaries. That day, Madeline was my last patient, and we were able to talk longer. She was by herself, away from her mother.

"How do you feel as a mother?" I began to test the field.

"I love it! It's strange, but I have more time for myself."

"And what do you do with that time?"

"I read; I write, and I can dream freely."

I didn't ask what was she reading or writing, but I did ask what she was dreaming about.

"I dream that one day I may fly away from this world."

"Why?"

"Because I can't find my place here! I feel like a caged bird!"

I looked at her frowning.

"Doctor, it's just a metaphoric flight! Don't worry! I want to ask you something more down to earth. Why doesn't my period come back?"

I explained to her that it was quite normal not to menstruate when breastfeeding, only she had to be careful if she didn't want to get pregnant again.

"That won't happen. At least not in this world!"

I figured out that when she was saying "this world" she was referring to the distorted world we were living in; had she said "in the other world" she would not have implied the after-life, but the world that was not accessible to us, due to politics and our lack of freedom.

Madeline didn't speak like an ordinary person. She used unexpected parables and metaphors that came out of her mouth as natural as everyday words. I watched her carefully and couldn't see any sign of depression. I have seen many women with postpartum depression after having given birth, with dysfunction that was not taken seriously during those days. I remembered their troubled, emptied looks quite well, when they should have been happy and fulfilled. It's true that many women had unwanted pregnancies because they had no other option, but even then, once the baby was born, their joy was overwhelming. Most of the deliveries were painful, too, natural, without much anesthesia, but the physical pain was always easily forgotten. If we didn't have such a short memory about pain, the human species would have been in great danger. Fortunately, with the first cry of the baby, the maternal instinct becomes stronger than anything else.

Nobody worried when a nursing woman looked sad. No psychiatrist had been called in to consult until the year when two women from the postpartum ward threw themselves through the fourth floor windows. The only solution the hospital administration came up with then was to install bars on those windows.

I could only see a bit of melancholy in Madeline's eyes, some sadness, desperation—regular symptoms that afflicted us all. Madeline was an artist at heart. A few years later, as I passed by a known bookstore in Bucharest, I saw her picture in the window. She was launching a book of poems. I entered the store and browsed through the book. The poems were profound, bringing to memory both Sorescu and Nichita, Romanian poets, but having a unique touch that could only come from the mind and soul of a woman. Even today I remember some of her lines. Since I'd last seen her, Madeline had become a student of literature and had won a prize for that book.

Then I forgot all about her. I saw her once on TV during the tormented first days of the Romanian Revolution when people were still killed in the streets. She spoke about poetry and how metaphors hid or spit out the truth. She was on TV, talking live, about our freedom, sitting on top of a tank in University Square with a loudspeaker in her hand, which she had pulled from the hands of some revolutionaries who'd lost their voices and their reason. For ten minutes Madeline's gentle voice dominated the crowd with unusual power and well controlled pathos.

A few days later I boarded a plane and left for the U.S. Most of the passengers were traumatized edgy Romanians who'd finally been allowed to fly away. They even smoked on the plane. We were all high, ready to explode. I arrived in New York with burnt wings, smelling of cheap freedom and cheaper cigarettes. Everything had suddenly become possible, and "the other world" was waiting for us. At least that's what we imagined. Before it was the Securitate that suspected us of wanting to leave the country, now a whole world suspected us of not wanting to go back.

At the American Consulate, one of the few buildings that wasn't touched by bullets, there was a huge line, but I had managed, after a few days of waiting, to get an American visa.

They weren't suspecting that a young gynecologist like me, with a wonderful future in a world that was just delivering itself through great pains of history would be crazy enough to stay in America, with no English, no recognized medical degree, and no rights to deliver women anymore.

Seventeen years later, I saw Madeline in New York. She wasn't a girl anymore, unsure if she'd even given birth, having trouble nursing, and wanting to fly away from the top of a Communist building. She had taken her flight and was a strong woman now, with wings opened wide. Madeleine became a known writer and was pregnant again. She'd come to speak at a conference at one of New York's universities, and I went to see her. She read a few of her new poems, already translated in other languages, and then interacted with the audience. She spoke good English. As I listened to her, I realized that our women, like many other women from Eastern Europe, have a particular combination of softness and femininity, always on the surface, mixed with a well-poised strength and power, nicely camouflaged somewhere in their reserve-arsenal. It's a combination that's hard to find in the Anglo-Saxon world. After the conference was over we met and she showed me a picture of her boy, now a grown man of more than six feet tall, her spitting image.

"Do you remember how scared I was that I was given someone else's baby? Those days..."

She had the same look in her eyes, although she'd changed a lot. She was a mature woman, stylish and balanced, who'd traveled more than I had, and seemed to know the world well. We had dinner together, and she told me that she had a few more weeks before she'd give birth again.

"How is your husband?" I asked her.

"Bogdan's father? He's fine, remarried. After I gave birth, our relationship didn't work any longer. It was my fault."

It was winter time and being dressed in layers, her pregnancy didn't show. She hadn't put on weight, and only the profile of her belly gave her away. She said that she'd be staying in the U.S. for a while and asked me if I could examine her in my office.

I saw her again after three days when she brought me her last two books. She was supple and joyful and looked like a pregnant model, only she had to give birth through caesarean again and that frightened her.

"I travel quite a lot, and I don't know when the labor pains will hit me."

I examined her and did an ultrasound that showed everything was fine. She was going to have a baby girl, but asked from the very beginning for me not to tell her the sex of the baby because she wanted to keep the mystery until birth, even though she didn't "know how to give birth." She was supposed to have the cesarean delivery in about three to four weeks if not sooner, so I said plainly: "Why don't you stay in New York? You have a sister in Queens, and I can deliver the baby in my hospital. Now, it isn't good for you to travel much." She seemed to be puzzled for a few seconds, and I continued. "Don't worry about the insurance. You can get some soon. Here, pregnant women are protected; moreover, the newborn baby will be an American by birthright. Many women want to give birth here just for that."

"Yes. It would be great if you could deliver my second baby 'in the other world,' as we dreamt back then!"

Every year I had few pregnant women: Romanian, Serbian or Russians, who would come to America just to give birth in the U.S.A. I had seen many pregnant women from all over the world brought in while in labor from J.F.K., taken by ambulance straight from a freshly landed plane. I told Madeline about one of these women who seem to have fallen from the sky. She was a Chinese woman who did not let anybody touch her or even get close to her bed. The woman, who already had a child in China, didn't have the right to have another one and was already six months pregnant with the second one when she'd left. She had run away from her province because she was afraid that her pregnancy would be discovered and she'd be taken by force to the hospital where the pregnancy would be terminated. Despite the gestational age, the fetus would be killed by injecting potassium into its heart. If the woman managed to give birth at home to a live child, she would have been severely fined, or the baby would have been taken and given up for adoption.

The Chinese woman, although in deep pain, did not allow anyone to examine her or even start an IV until an interpreter was finally found.

"You said that the woman had fallen from the sky? That's a beautiful metaphor," said Madeline, as if speaking about herself.

By the end of our dinner, she seriously considered delivering her baby in New York and had agreed to come to the hospital the next day. I was 'on-call' and I wanted to show her the hospital which has a new "state of the art" wing for obstetrics.

The next day, she stepped shyly into the hospital and told me a few times that hospitals scared her with all that went on inside their walls. I tried to make her relax and took her to the Delivery Room which happened to be quiet at the time. Every door we were going through would automatically open after my finger prints were checked and recognized. It was a new security system that had been introduced not long before, now considered standard in the U.S. Sometimes I had to scan my thumb a couple of times before the machine would recognize my fingerprints. I wasn't fond of those doors that kept opening one after another. Since the new system had been introduced, it had become harder to roam through the hospital.

One of the doors refused to open, and Madeline and I got stuck in a hallway until a nurse showed up.

"Why is there so much security?" Madeline asked uneasily, stressing the word "Security".

"So that nobody can steal a newborn. The little ones have an electronic chip attached to their legs which would shut the doors. Nor can the babies be exchanged by mistake, because we have all kinds of methods to identify them. Be sure, babies won't escape from here!"

"Who would want to steal a newborn baby?" she asked me in a stupor.

I just shrugged my shoulders. Then I showed her the Operating Rooms, perfectly isolated, anti-septic; all the other rooms had A.C. and sealed windows that could never be opened.

"Not even a bird can escape this place," I quipped. Madeline was looking at me rather scared. When we left, we had to pass through the same doors.

"Very nice and 'safe', indeed!" she said when we parted. But it's too much; it's like a beautiful prison."

She called the next day to thank me and said she had decided to fly back to her country.

"I think it's better to return to my birdcage… Keep your fingers crossed for me!"

She'd chosen to give birth in our old city where the new hospital had new windows installed and the doors opened and closed the old fashioned way.

HIND END FIRST

ALL THE INFORMATION COMING from the ambulance driver rushing to the hospital didn't make much sense: they were bringing a thirty-five-year-old woman, having her second baby, who'd just tried to give birth at home with a midwife. She was found in her bedroom with a half- born baby coming out of her womb. Or with the other half not yet born, depending how you look at it. The baby was trying to get out with his hind end first; meaning a breech delivery.

My first reaction to such information was one of disbelief. I asked myself almost instinctually where in hell we were on the planet and what millennium were we living in? Who would try to deliver a baby at home, in a bedroom—a baby that was coming out hind end first? In New York City in the Twenty-First Century?!

We had no time to ask ourselves useless questions because the EMT's had brought the woman in on a stretcher and had taken her straight into the Operating Room where everything had been prepared. The baby's pelvis was completely out, the membranes already ruptured by one of the brave midwives who'd tried to deliver her at home, and one of the baby's legs was dangling between the mother's legs. It was one of the largest newborn legs that I have ever seen. The other leg was still inside the mother's pelvis, stretched along the boy's body. That was what kept the boy inside, still safe in his shelter.

We were two of us Attendings 'on-call', and took turns with the admissions. This case went to my colleague who'd just finished his Residency. He told me frankly that he had never assisted a breech delivery. "Frank Breech," gave his name to such a presentation of the baby struggling to come out. In the States, any mother who is experiencing a baby in breech position and goes into labor must deliver by caesarean because it's considered a dangerous birth. The woman was accompanied by two midwives, the same who'd delivered her first born at home. They looked scared to death and swore that the boy had been in a cranial position, but had suddenly turned with his hind end first just before his appearance, like a funny juggler doing an impermissible obstetric trick. That all happened after the poor woman had been screaming for a couple of hours. I've never heard such improbable idiocy, and the first to react were our own midwives who told them that it was better if they too shut up, waited outside, and prayed.

Stella, one of the midwives with whom I'd worked for years, knew right away what she had to do. She took a sterile towel and kept the baby's bottom blocked where it was. Judging by the size of the leg, the baby was very large.

In Romania I'd assisted many breech deliveries. There weren't too many regulations during the '80s, nor was there a fear of lawsuits. Anyhow, a baby of that size wouldn't have been allowed to be delivered naturally even in Romania.

They all looked at me to see what I was doing. I told Stella to keep the baby tight inside, as best as she could. Stella, a strong woman, looked like a rugby player ready to ram the pack. Had the baby tried to come down a little further, he would have tried to breathe instinctively and most likely would have choked to death because he had no air in his mom's womb.

I asked for a portable ultrasound, and in between the mother's wriggling and screaming, I tried to see the position of the baby's head, which was still up inside the mother's uterus. Like I thought, it was a very large head, completely flipped and deflected backwards with the back of the head touching the spine, as if he was trying to get a glimpse of the sky through his mother's womb. I was pondering what to do, in order for him not to stay in that critical position for too long. He had his arms raised above his head which would have made a vaginal delivery much worse. I'd never been in such a situation before, not even back in Romania.

Getting over the outrage that had overwhelmed me, I tried to handle things as they were. It wasn't hard to imagine what would have happened had I left the baby to continue its way out with his hind end first, as it would have been quite normal in that situation. I knew that I'd have had big problems to deliver the head after the rest of the body. In such a case, I'd have to get one of my hands into the uterus and pull down his hands which were now over his head, then find the baby's mouth, get two fingers inside, and by pushing hard at the base of the tongue on its mandibular, try to move the baby's head from its awkward position and somehow pull it out. It was a difficult and dangerous maneuver to do on such a large baby. Add to that, everything had to be done fast otherwise the baby could have quickly been suffocated in our hands. A nightmare for any obstetrician.

I looked at Stella, who was on all fours trying to ease the baby's exit. I explained to the mother in a few words that if we just waited for the baby to come out we might not be able to pull its head out in time. I didn't mention that I'd seen a similar case in my country, when a poor woman, who didn't want to give birth at home, was brought in to the hospital too late. Not only did the baby die, but we cracked its skull in the end, and the baby's head had to be removed separately with instruments that American hospitals have not kept on hand for decades. That procedure was called a craniotomy, and the baby's head would be crushed in order to be extracted, thus saving the mother. I told her that as a last ditch scenario, a desperate caesarean would give us a better chance of saving the baby.

"Desperate?"

Yes, desperate, because half of the baby was already out.

I quickly asked her if she knew that the baby was coming with its hind end first, or whether she'd been seen by a doctor, or if she'd had an ultrasound before.

No, nobody had done any such thing, because she wanted it all to be "natural," meaning she didn't want to have anything to do with a clinic or with a doctor. The woman gave me a strange and empty look.

"Do what you know is best!" she said.

I didn't know anything about her. I could only see that she was an educated woman, who most likely worked in Manhattan, maybe in a law firm, and who wanted to give birth at home for her own private reasons. I could only guess her rationale, although it was hard for me to understand it. This woman was afraid of doctors! When I spoke to her, she had the same fearful look on her face as the women in Communist Romania did, during the times when abortions were entirely forbidden. Women who had abortions were called "criminals" and would come to the hospital only when there was no other choice, other than to have us, doctors, finish a job that had been started by someone else, illegally, in dangerous circumstances. Now we didn't have the police on our tails, nor was there a Securitate; there was only our own consciousness, and of course the lawyers, a sophisticated system that promoted fear, made to not only frighten doctors, but also frighten patients.

Why would a woman want to give birth at home, "naturally," dangerously, on the edge, when on each corner of New York City a hospital waited for them? Why are they afraid of doctors and hospitals? Truth be told, the rate of caesarean deliveries has reached 50% or more in some areas. We live in a system where no error is accepted, no negative outcome, even when nature itself pushes things that way. We now have conferences mourning the disappearance of the obstetrical art in America and highlighting so many maneuvers and procedures that can be avoided today by doing a simple caesarean, an operation that's being done with greater and greater ease. These procedures, that nobody will know how to perform, will remain only as historical relics in a few obstetrical books. Any physician who's been in an American court at least one time can better understand why we've gotten here.

That night I asked Stella to stay still and keep the baby inside. I walked out to scrub with my younger colleague.

"How should we get this baby out?" he asked.

"I have no clue, but we will somehow!"

My colleague was visibly more stressed than I was. The case was under his name, but mine also, because I'd gotten myself fully involved. If the case was brought to trial, we would go hand in hand to the Queens Civil Court, the imposing building that could be seen from our hospital.

The two midwives who assisted the woman at home suddenly relaxed. The anesthesiologist put the woman to sleep, and I opened her belly as fast as I could. The lower part of the uterus was so dilated that it was ready to burst, which would have happened soon had the woman continued to push. I did a classical incision on the uterus, from top to bottom and opened the uterus wide, like a book. I felt Stella breathing under the operating field, our wonderful midwife who was holding the baby in.

Stella was originally from Scotland and spoke English with a strong accent which I loved. In her younger years, she'd seen plenty of dramas from where she came from. She loved her profession and loved America, although "the bloody bastards" asked her to take an English proficiency test, in line with all the other foreigners.

I got inside the uterus with one hand and tried to get it up around the head of the baby, but his hands were kept up as if holding his head. I managed to pull a hand down without breaking any bones and got into the baby's mouth. I flexed the head and pulled it out after enlarging the cut. Then I grabbed the baby and pulled him quickly out.

"Make sure you don't pull me with him," joked Stella from under the table.

The baby recovered in a few minutes and did well. He was fourteen pounds and had a sad and frightened look on his face, keeping his eyes wide open as if he'd been taken by absolute surprise. A newborn usually keeps his eyes closed because, for him, there's suddenly too much light, even if he doesn't seem to see it. In the hour that followed, we had to repair the uterus which was bleeding profusely. We did the sutures rapidly, and we ordered a large amount of blood from the blood bank, the only bank where we had an open line of credit, day or night. We massaged the uterus, injected it with all kinds of strong medication, which usually helped, but the over abused uterus continued to bleed and remain flaccid. I tied both uterine arteries, this being the last maneuver before we were to move to a hysterectomy. She had lost lots of blood. I was terrified thinking that the woman was asleep and that the whole drama was going to happen without a proper consent being signed. I asked my colleague, the Resident, and the rest of the team that was hanging around, but nobody seemed to know if a proper consent had been signed by the woman.

"We're in trouble," said my colleague. His face was covered by a surgical mask, but I could see his frightened guilty look, as if the two of us had created the whole drama. Only after I managed to tie the arteries, which were bringing blood to the uterus, could we breathe easier because that stopped the bleeding. We decided that hemostasis was good enough and we could close her up. When we finally got to the abdominal wall, I left the room. I was entirely drenched in sweat as if after a sauna, and I went to the locker room to change clothes. The two midwives were contrite in the waiting room and were talking to the husband. I tried to avoid them, and they seemed to avoid me too. It was a fourteen-pound baby they all tried to delivered at home, a baby who had turned himself upside down with his hind end first, at the last moment! That was way too much! I refused to believe that story that defied common sense and any law of physics. The husband approached me and asked if everything was all right. I asked again whether his wife had been seen by a doctor before birth. No, she hadn't been seen by any doctor, because she had avoided doctors as much as she could. Her pregnancy had only been monitored by the two midwives who'd listened to the baby's heart, checked her blood pressure, and asked his wife if she took her vitamins. Everything had gone well, according to them, until the baby "flipped over" and unexpectedly pushed one leg out.

"Doctor, I saw it with my own eyes," the father said.

Blood rushed to my head again, and I tried not to say a word. In the end, I told him that his wife should have seen a doctor at least once before term and should have been scheduled for a caesarean from the beginning.

"Doctor, my wife doesn't believe in caesareans!" he said.

I closed my eyes and saw stars.

"OK, Thank God, your boy and your wife are fine. Congratulations!" And I left for the locker room.

There are women who don't believe in caesareans, as if a caesarean is a new concept, a new unorthodox philosophy that must be shunned. I often heard women who had unplanned pregnancies saying that they would not terminate because they "do not believe in abortions." That, I could easily understand. Refusing abortions is associated with religious beliefs; but caesareans? The truth is that when I started working in the States, I'd been startled myself because the caesarean rate was 25%. Since then, the index had moved up to double that.

For a doctor coming from Romania where the rate of caesareans was only 6%, this rate looked like an obstetrical trip into the future. I knew that in Brooklyn there were delivery units without doctors, where everything was performed by midwives. The idea of going back to "natural" became a power play of sorts.

One of my patients walked out of my office rather upset when I recommended a cesarean delivery because she was carrying a ten-pound baby and had a small pelvis. She took her file and moved to a clinic with midwives. She delivered by caesarean, only after she'd been through twenty-four hours of horrible labor and she finally had to be taken to the closest hospital. Another lady pregnant with a baby just as big, but at age forty-one, wanted to give birth under water. I saw her in postpartum and she told me about her subaquatic adventure that ended in the Operating Room but only after she'd bloodied the bath tub where she tried to deliver her baby. I have nothing against these types of deliveries, but when a patient asked me if I believed in belly dancing exercises and belly dancing during labor, I felt it was too much for me.

I checked the Internet site of one of those clinics that advertised this type of dance practice to help bring the baby down through a woman's narrow pelvis, and they were offering training that came with a specialist who was supposed to lead the show. I had the faint impression that before my retirement I was going to see that kind of performance. That night, when I left the Operating Room looking at the two adventurous midwives, I remembered an old French comedy with Louis de Funès: two weird nuns running wild, driving the monastery car, getting themselves into all kinds of dangerous and hilarious trouble.

Now that the problem had been solved, the midwives seemed to be completely relaxed. Only the whole affair wasn't going to stop there. As soon as I got undressed and ready to take a shower, my beeper went off.

"You've got to come back. They have a problem with the final counting," said Stella gravely, meaning the counting of the instruments and materials we used during surgery.

If the mother and child were "counted" correctly, plus the instruments and all the operating materials came out fine, then what was wrong with the "counting"? "Counting correct" is what I had heard one of the nurses say before I threw out my gloves. When I went back, the counting process was still ongoing because something was evidently missing. One unmarked 4x4 inch gauze sponge, which had been opened in a hurry by one of the nurses, could not be accounted for. We searched everywhere, even under the patient, and then followed the protocol and asked Radiology to come in and do an X-ray. The four-inch square gauze was rather visible on the woman's pelvis. Being unmarked with a radiopaque plastic, could have been easily mistaken as one made of special fibrin fibers which I purposely placed there to stop the bleeding. Nobody had said a word.

In the meantime, the Chief Resident, as instructed, called the Chairman. I explained to him that I believed the foreign body was just the pellicle of fibrin. Only the hospital protocol said clearly: the patient cannot be taken off the operating table until everything is counted out. I took a cotton gauze and checked it against the fibrin one. They looked pretty much the same. I ran to Radiology and asked the technician to do an X-ray of my hands. Bob, the six-foot-eight giant from Long Island, muscular and full of tattoos, was just getting back to his nap on the stretcher with his knees bent. At my request, he answered with a strange look: "Are you serious, doc?"

"C'mon Bob. We have no time to waste. The patient is on the table." I placed the cotton gauze in one of my hands and the fibrin sheet on the other to see how they would be seen on an X- ray. The cotton gauze was visible but the fibrin wasn't, while my hands looked wider than I expected.

"Congratulations, Doctor. You don't have any osteoporosis," said Bob.

We had to re-open the patient's abdomen and search through her belly for a 4 x 4-inch gauze which could have been anywhere. Even worse, she could have started to bleed again. That was what I feared most. The Chief Resident looked over the Internet with the Chairman in a search of that darn fibrin sheet which was invisible, radiologically speaking. In the meantime, everybody was turning the whole operating room upside down but the gauze refused to appear. The smile on those two midwives' faces had disappeared again. They didn't look like the cheerful French nuns any more. Meanwhile I scrubbed ready to get back and continue the operation. The Chief Resident came running in and told me that the Chairman wanted to talk to me. He got hold of one of the producers of that fibrin pellicle who told him that their product may become visible at X-ray if there are air bubbles trapped inside the abdomen after closing. I took a deep breath, threw away my gloves, and asked the anesthesiologist to wake the patient up.

It was five o'clock in the morning and made no sense for me to lie down on a bed. I finally went into the shower, bathed and changed the scrubs which were stinking with acid perspiration that only stress or fear can stir up. I went back, and until the new shift showed up, chatted with Stella and the Residents.

One of our own midwives told us that she had given birth to both of her children at home, but at least she had ultrasounds done and was seen by an obstetrician during her pregnancy. So the fear of caesareans was that great that even our own midwives were giving birth at home! I also found out that the midwife who had assisted her deliveries had received $8,000 out of the $8,600 from the insurance company that she had billed, and in the end, the new mom got a separate bill for $600, which drove her mad. For the caesarean we did that night, we would receive something between $600 and $1000. The hospital charge would go up to $20,000. The insurance companies obviously preferred to see babies being born at home.

Before I left the hospital I went to see the big baby. The leg that had come out first was still swollen. The boy was sleeping quietly, and his chubby face had the strange expression of a slightly troubled grown man who had not yet figured out all that had happened to him. When I tried to hold his hands, I saw that in one of them, he triumphantly squeezed a 4 x 4-inch piece of gauze.

ZODIACS, SIGNS AND BELIEFS

WHEN I WAS STILL WAITING in my mother's womb, my parents were young teachers in a remote Romanian village. It was December 1953, and I'm sure they didn't care what kind of horoscope sign would hang over my head after I came out. Back then, nobody cared about horoscopes, signs, or zodiacs. Everybody assumed that astrology was forbidden, just as religion was, or other beliefs that could keep us tied to an obscure bourgeois past which had to be erased and completely forgotten. It was the time of the most radical and destructive Romanian Communism. On top of that came the coldest winter since the end of World War II, but people were much more afraid of the Communist terror than of nature's whims. Any adult could be arrested over night, declared an enemy of the State, and then disappeared for no particular reason. Only small children and the unborn, like me, were considered pure and not guilty.

A heavy snowfall blocked most roads; the temperature dropped below minus 20 degrees Celsius, and life came to a scary standstill, including those four to five ambulances, leftovers from the war, that served the whole county of Bistrita. My mother had little prenatal care from the local doctor. He listened once or twice to my heart using a sort of funnel and advised her to eat well and stay warm at home. He also told her that she would deliver me around Christmas, or New Year's Eve, to be precise. There was a midwife in the village, but with such weather, there was little hope she could get to our house.

When my mother went into labor, my father panicked. Running and sliding, he got to the post office and called an ambulance from Bistrita, a city that was fourteen miles away, where there was a maternity ward and three doctors. The simple fact that the ambulance arrived in less than five hours, eight years after the war, during a time when my grandfather was stigmatized because he was seen as a former bourgeoisie and my father had been imprisoned by the Communist regime for almost a year, makes me think in retrospect, that we still lived in a world with traces of discipline and organization, even some human compassion. I, the one on his way into that new world, was assumed to be crystal clear in body and soul, still uncontaminated by any ideology or belief—raw material for the future.

My grandparents and great-grandparents from my mother's side were all alive and waiting for my arrival. Their longevity was impressive. They were stubborn survivors in between centuries, empires, and social orders. We would later say that they lived so long because they didn't have stress. They went through two world wars and the beginning of Communism. My parents, who had survived the Second World War carried the hardship of Communism on their shoulders from its beginning to its end. We were the new-comers, "the baby-boomers," the generation that invented "stress" and immortality.

The ambulance had chains on its wheels, but still skidded badly somewhere between Barla and Marisel, two villages where my chromosomes from my mother's side had survived for centuries. Later, countless times, my father showed me the curve in the road and the ditch where I'd been almost born at minus 25 degrees Celsius, and the house of the man who saved me by pulling a pair of oxen from his stable and managing to drag the ambulance out of the ditch. Because of the darkness, extreme emotions, or because of Communism which did not believe in anything, nobody would remember the exact day and time of my birth. Even though the steeple of the German cathedral in Bistrita always showed the exact time, and its bell had been ringing hourly for about four centuries, nobody had the time and initiative to document such details. Still nobody knows if my birth was on December 30th or 31st, or the exact hour. Therefore, I only know that I'm a Capricorn, according to the European horoscope, and a Snake by the Chinese one. No other details matter. My ascendant sign, which is based on the hour of your birth, will remain a mystery—no big deal to me.

I became curious about my signs only after I moved to America, when I reached a very low point in my life and went through some strange experiences that were difficult to grasp or explain. By chance I met a few zodiac experts (and there are plenty) who tried to find explanations for the experiences I was going through based on my birth signs. I did not believe such things, but I browsed the Chinese and European zodiacs, read about the signs of some close friends and family members, and realized that there might be a grain of truth in astrology. It was similar to that plum kernel that Transylvanian people put in their traditional brandy, called Tzuica, which can change its taste dramatically. There is no doubt that we are born between the moon, the sun, and many other stars, which move above our heads and whose alignment at the time of our birth probably influences our personality, temperament, or even destiny. Maybe that is why we are so different from each other, yet so similar in so many ways.

I still remember my mother's perplexed reaction when, over the phone, I asked her certain details of my birth. Her only memory of that event was that it was a horrible experience. I persisted and talked to my father whom I pressured with questions about the exact time I was born. An American friend of mine was trying to do my horoscope, and she couldn't believe that a man like me, coming from a European country, had no one in my family who could remember what time their only son was born. On the other hand, my sudden and stupid questions worried my parents a lot, and they asked me straight out if I was still in my right mind. It was around 1990, and I was struggling as a recent immigrant in the U.S. My parents were living in a very confused, unstable, post-Communist Romania, but suggested that it might be better if I went back home to the land where my "signs" were originally conceived.

My birth eventually turned into a public lie. My mother remained in the hospital for almost a week due to complications, while I was quite blue and spent a few days in an incubator. And so, my father went to the town hall and registered my birth day as January 1st. He did that in order to help me skip a year and eventually spared me the mandatory military service when I turned eighteen. This proved to be a useful little maneuver which had no repercussions on my zodiac sign.

My second birth in America was a gradual one, way more traumatizing than my biological one. Some people think there should be a special horoscope for immigrants but now I don't care much about my zodiac signs. Last time I had a chance to clarify my zodiac was a few years ago when my father called to congratulate me on my birthday. My mother was lying in bed, having been paralyzed for the last four years. One of her legs had been amputated but she continued to feel as if it was there, although her mind was clear to the end. She used to say that her lost leg was an envoy sent on a mission to the other side. My father put her on the phone and she asked: "Do you still want to know when exactly you were born?" I was surprised that she still remembered that awkward detail. I visited every year, spending two or three days with them, holding her hand and talking to her. Otherwise we were on the phone weekly. I sent them money and my encouragement from America.

One day, early on a May morning, my sister called and told me that our mother had passed away in her sleep. The ambulance may have come faster that time, but my father hadn't called it. Before she fell asleep, she'd watched *Dallas,* as usual, her preferred soap opera, which she'd been watching for the last twenty years.

In 1993, when I came to visit from the U.S.A. for the first time, we had a very emotional reunion. We hadn't seen each other for over three years. I was going through an immigration nightmare, a painful transition between systems. When I arrived from the airport, mother hugged me in tears, held me a few moments, put some food on a plate, then simply said: "Now please excuse me, because *Dallas* is starting." Soon, we were eating and watching TV as if I'd never left.

In Romania, medicine was considered to be almost an art, while in the U.S. it is seen as an exact science. Today, every hospital in the world records the date, hour, and minute of a child's birth, along with the newborn's Apgar score. Doctors don't get involved in astrology and zodiac issues; they only care about the Apgar score which can predict quite exactly the fate, health, and the immediate well-being of a newborn. Medicine had to find a common denominator and language in order to establish a universal scientific basis that explains the state of a newborn child, and then to scientifically record that state. About fifty years ago, while she worked at Columbia-Presbyterian Hospital in New York City, Doctor Virginia Apgar introduced this famous score which bears her last name. It is now used everywhere and has led to a spectacular decrease in perinatal mortality. The score is based upon the newborn's breathing rate, its movements and heartbeat, the color and muscular tonus of the baby, recorded at a minute and then five minutes after its birth. A score of 8 or higher is good, while a 2 or 3 Apgar is frightening.

"Tell me what Apgar score you had, and I'll know who you are," joked a former colleague of mine, a neonatologist.

If one happens to be sued for the death or injury of a newborn, the first thing that each party wants to know is the child's Apgar score. It can even predict the development of a human being in the near future. There are also scores that measure pain on a scale from 1 to 10, although it's difficult to estimate pain correctly. Such measuring systems, related to these particular problems, are very sought-after in the medical field, in order to come up with universal standards for issues related to health and illness. How sad or how happy are you on scale from 1 to 10?

Astrology and zodiacs are as old as religions and seem to gain in popularity and stir up more curiosity. The Chinese have always been the champions of believing in signs under which we are born, although they still live under a Communist regime, a restrictive ideology. Forced by government politics to have only one child, with great care, Chinese families choose the year they will procreate for the one and only time in their lives. Therefore, in China more children are born during the year of the Dragon or Tiger than during any other years whose signs are less popular. Such years have very low birth rates. When it comes to your future child, everything can be controlled, including gender.

In my hospital in New York, I see women from the remotest parts of the world. With pregnancy and birth, some carry with them old customs, rituals, beliefs and superstitions. Moreover, they mix their native habits with the ones in their adopted land. In British Guyana, the Indian Hindu, who went there as free people, mixed their beliefs with voodoo practices kept by the African slaves. Guyanese men cannot see their newborn until after their priest, called a Pandith, checks the child's zodiac and the signs under which he is born. I have no clue how he does that. One of these men didn't see his newborn son for three days, until their Pandith came back from vacation. He carefully checked the baby and ceremoniously announced to them, for a fee, that his boy was born under the best signs possible. Otherwise he was supposed to fix the signs for another fee, to smoothen the boy's way in his new life.

The Vietnamese people have their own customs. After a birth, they claim a piece of the child's umbilical cord. When the baby is out and placed on the mother's abdomen, American midwives encourage the father to cut the cord himself. This is somehow an American custom which surprised me at the beginning, because I'd never seen men participating in the process. Some men refuse to cut the umbilical cord. One of them, too emotional, almost cut his finger with the scissors shaking in his hand. That Vietnamese man eventually succeeded in cutting the cord; then he cut it one more time and quickly put the piece in his pocket. Our midwife ended up so scandalized that she called for the head nurse to investigate. That ritual was not included in the hospital protocol or in any New York State legislation.

In American hospitals all religions are accepted with no restriction. Just across from my hospital there is one of the largest mosques in New York. Half of our Muslim patients are named Kaur, the other half Begun, originally from Pakistan and Bangladesh. They do not want male doctors to treat their wives, but when there are only two male doctors 'on-call' they have no choice. The midwife does everything, while we try to negotiate with the husband who guards the door to allow us in, if an emergency should arise.

For years, I have seen Rabbi Steiner wandering through the hospital. At the beginning I thought that he was one of the old time doctors who supervises the Interns and Residents, until one of his relatives came to deliver her baby while I was 'on-call.' Rabbi Steiner wore an old fashioned black double-breasted suit and a hat which made him look a bit like Al Capone. He simply told me: "I'm the hospital Rabbi. The girl is my niece and I'll hang around until the baby is out." He had a hospital ID. It was a Saturday and our "Jewish elevator" was set to stop automatically at every floor, because the people from the nearby religious community were not supposed to push the elevator's buttons during Shabbat. I had a long chat with the Rabbi, whose ancestors were originally from Bucovina, part of Romania. Now his congregation is mixed with believers from all over the world. While we were talking in the corridor, his relative delivered her seventh baby in bed, silently, without pushing, screaming, or moaning.

Rabbi Steiner brushed his shoulder scattered with dandruff, shook my hand, and left, telling me with serenity: "Doctor, God sometimes solves problems by himself!"

I knew the hospital priest well. Father Gregor was a tall man, always in his black suit, with a hard-white collar around his neck. I've never seen him in the Labor and Delivery Unit. At Christmas parties, he says a prayer and blesses our gathering in a way that won't let you guess if he's a Catholic, Protestant or any other denomination. In his hospital chapel anybody can pray to any God in any way, even Jehovah Witnesses, who still scare me a lot with their categorical refusal to accept blood transfusions. I did surgery and cesarean sections on some of them, and their own hospital protocol is damn clear: no blood transfusions even if they die on the operating table...

I was recently discussing the date we should schedule the delivery of her baby with one of my pregnant Eastern European patients. She was about eight months pregnant, and we were talking about her third caesarian delivery which should be performed after thirty-nine weeks of gestation. She wanted to know the exact date of the caesarian well in advance in order to bring her mother over from Romania at the right time. But she had another reason. She had given birth to her first two boys through caesarian section too. I don't remember the reason for her first caesarian, but the first intervention of this kind brings up the second, then the third one, and so on. There are women who deliver up to five, even six children through caesarian section.

With the scheduled caesarean deliveries there comes the time when you, as the doctor, have to calculate the due date, which is a pretty simple process. You go straight to the computer or grab that "wheel of fortune," a present from a pharmaceutical company, which identifies when the pregnancy will reach forty weeks, which is the accepted due date. I had decided to take the baby out on a Wednesday, which worked very well for me since I was scheduled to be 'on-call' that day. But the woman begged me to wait until Friday or Saturday, which brought up some real risks because she could go into labor and the newborn would have to be delivered immediately. Still, her argument won over mine. That Thursday marked the beginning of a new zodiac sign, Leo, a better and more prosperous one, and my patient strongly believed in astrological signs. She had carefully planned all her previous pregnancies, therefore her other two children were also Leos, just like her husband. I tried to convince her that so many Leos in her house might be too much to handle, but I couldn't change her mind.

"It's the best sign, doctor. If you take the baby out around noon, it will be even better because the child's ascendant will be under the Leo sign too. Can you do this for my baby? Please!"

I swallowed, nodded in kind of an agreement, and scheduled her for the requested day.

I was left with a bitter taste and an undefined sensation of guilt. I really asked myself if there was any truth in these beliefs. Was there any way that we, modern obstetricians, could change astrological signs by changing birth times? Maybe even the destiny of so many children? That thought gave me strange chills because I knew that I had no divine qualifications. Not that I wanted them either!

The story kept haunting me, and that night I had a dream—a real nightmare. In it I was on the Labor and Delivery Ward, which was crowded with women in active labor. All twelve Delivery Rooms, and we really had twelve, were named for the zodiac signs: the room of Leo, Sagittarius, Capricorn,

Pisces etc. Under each name was written the Chinese sign which belonged to the year. Every single room was full of pregnant women wanting to deliver as soon as possible.

Followed by two strong tall Residents, I was doing the rounds. We were going from room to room and reluctantly asking every woman what sign she wanted for her baby. We were all wearing photo ID's with our names, the zodiac signs, and the ascendant sign under which we were born. Only on mine was written "person without known ascendant." The head nurse was named Paolina, a nurse from Romania, who in the old days had been a Police and Securitate collaborator. We all feared her. In my dream, Paolina was leading the whole show, carefully supervising what I was doing. She was wearing a large white helmet and was directing traffic in the L&D unit using a big stick. To the undecided women, she was harshly ordering them to choose, because this was now part of the state politics and even nature itself. She was shouting mercilessly and writing down everything in a big notebook. She completely ignored all the computers around her and slammed them with her stick as she passed by. Curiously enough, I had no regrets about the computers. It was a real nightmare. In my dream I was talking in English, Spanish, using short expressions in Russian, Polish, Bengali and Urdu, exactly as I do in real life. Then nurses began moving the pregnant women into the room they chose, and after delivery, gave them birth certificates, already printed with the proper zodiac sign. At some point, my real patient showed up in labor, terrified, and whispered in my ear that she gave up her Leo request and no longer wanted that particular sign anymore. I tried to put her in a room with no signs, but nurse Paolina saw me and took a whack at us with her stick, shouting that we couldn't do that. We had entered an orderly well managed world, where nothing was left to flow freely. Infuriated, she told me that astrology was now part of the new doctrine, just like dialectic materialism was a mandatory discipline studied in medical schools. It's time to understand, damn it! At this moment, thank God, I woke up! I was sweating and panting like a racing horse who'd had to jump some imaginary obstacles. I was happy that all of it was just a stupid nightmare; then I took a shower and went to my sign-less hospital. The following night, well after midnight, I was called back to full reality by the husband of my astrologically obsessed patient who sounded like a worried Leo: "My wife's water broke."

I went to the hospital where my patient was in active labor, having strong and painful contractions. The OR was busy with another caesarean delivery that had just begun. I started to worry because my patient's uterus, already cut twice, could rupture if we waited too long. I asked for another anesthesiologist but I knew that would take some time until he arrived from home. It was a night with a full moon, and in every delivery room, there was a woman in labor. My patient's pain got stronger but I could do nothing without an anesthesiologist. The patient's husband, otherwise a calm man, became nervous, the agitation aggravating him even more. From the next delivery room, we heard strange feminine voices, incantations, and even some drums and bizarre instruments, which puzzled me.

"What's going on there, doctor?"

I walked into that room to see what was happening, hoping to help because the night team was clearly overwhelmed with problems. In the room, a 16-year-old girl was just delivering, and the noise was being made by five massive women from Brooklyn. They were all nicely dressed wearing colorful skirts and large straw-hats as black women from the South wear for Sunday gospel. They were loudly praying to the Lord. I imagined them in their churches in the Bronx, singing and praying in a crescendo as the baby's head started to show. The young girl, numbed with morphine, was hardly pushing, trying, in a trance to keep the pace with the women around her. Then the baby's head came out and the chorus and the tambourine became apocalyptic. "*Thank you, Jesus! Praise you Lord! Halleluiah, Hallelujah!*"

In the meantime, the anesthesiologist showed up and we finally got my patient into the Operating Room.

"What are those women doing there?" the scared, pale, husband asked me.

"They're praying!"

When I opened his wife's abdomen, the uterus already had a small rupture and through the membranes I could see the baby's face. Then I got a big surprise: it was a girl, not a boy, screaming at the top of her lungs. I completely forgot the mother and her husband who were holding hands under the covering sheets as I heard my patient's voice calling me in Romanian:

"Doctor, doctor, my husband passed out!"

I looked over those sheets and saw the man flat on the floor, paper-white, out of this world. The rest of the procedure went quietly, but the whole team was freaking out because they also had to take care of her husband. He remained lying down while a female student splashed him with water and reassured him that everything was just fine. He kept telling her: "I'm a sensitive man, madam! It was too much for me!"

In the morning I ordered a CAT scan for him just to be sure he had no head trauma. Their girl was crying loudly, and not because she was born a Cancer. Her mother told me happily that Cancer was a very good sign for girls. In the end, they were all happy because subconsciously they'd wanted a girl to add some astrological variety to their house. Next, I saw her in her postpartum room. There were all men in there and they asked me to take a picture with them. Her husband had a bump on his head and was seriously wondering how in the world I could do that kind of job day-in-and-day-out.

His wife hesitantly asked me: "I could see from your office diplomas that you're a Capricorn! May I ask, at what hour of the day were you born?" I looked at her for a while and answered like a man who doesn't know where he's coming from, but might know where he's going—"At 2:30 in the morning, madam!"

A LUCKY WOMAN

I HAVE A GREAT understanding of scars, those marks that will stay with us forever, that unlike tattoos, we try to hide. In time, we get used to our scars and don't care anymore, like we do with some tattoos made during uninspired moments of our existence. I have a few old wounds myself, healed for quite some time, and I'm quite fed up telling their stories when somebody looks at my body on the beach and asks me with concern:

"Ouch! Where did you get that big scar under your arm? How about this one on your chest?"

"Of course, they're from duels with my own immigration, with American imperialism. Swashbuckling duels I won in the end," I'd say.

Everybody knows nowadays that most scars are made in the Operating Room, done by doctors who had to get into our bodies in order to fix something. Every day I see lots of scars (even more tattoos) and ask my patients how they got them. Some are obvious, as those from caesarians, appendectomies or cholecystectomies, done before the laparoscopy era. Breasts have scars left by operations made to remove benign tumors or cancers, scars which now are getting smaller and smaller.

In the U.S., any gynecological examination should start with the breasts. This is one peculiar reason why some strange people envy us. When I least expect it, I could be hit with a ridiculous comment which curbs my appetite for the conversation. It's true, we examine breasts every day and we have to do it because it's necessary and because, why not say it, the women's breasts are the most common reason for malpractice lawsuits in the States. Breast cancer is one of the most frequent cancers in women, and the New York City area has the highest rate in the world. Despite that, many women do not want their breasts examined and refuse to have a mammography, an examination some consider akin to torture.

I have to admit that I forgot why Miss M. came to see me in the office. She was quite reluctant to allow me to examine her breasts. She let me do it only after I told her that breast cancer genes could be genetically transmitted. Her mother had died of breast cancer. She shyly took off her bra and only then did I understand why she was so reluctant to show me her chest. Her breasts were full of strange scars, healed in a bizarre way that surgically didn't make any sense to me. I hadn't seen anything like that before so automatically I asked her where her scars came from.

"From a knife!" she said simply.

"You mean a scalpel?"

"No, a kitchen knife…" A long pause followed, while I almost forgot why we were there.

"A former lover of mine! I was very young and used to work in Galati's old metallurgic plant in Romania. Perhaps you've heard of it? I was living in one of those dormitories made for singles," she continued embarrassed.

"But why did he do it?"

"Jealousy, passion, I suppose! I almost died."

Yes, I've heard about that famous metallurgic plant, Communist Industrial Romania's pride, now closed, taken apart and partially hauled to India as scrap metal. Thousands of young workers lived crowded in small Communist buildings, working 24-hour shifts, eating in dark cantinas, drinking vodka, loving each other in tight spaces that brought so many to despair and alcoholism. But still, what had that metallurgic conglomerate to do with her botched breasts, now full of scars? Why would a man of any nature, in any kind of world, do something so awful to a woman? What kind of passion and craziness could create such cruelty?

I raised my eyes and carefully looked at Miss M., who was, I would say, a rather simple, ordinary woman, who otherwise wouldn't have caught my eye. Older than thirty-five, tall, and a bit plump, she was now shaped by the American food she ate in the last six to seven years at the Romanian restaurant where she worked as a waitress. Her eyes were dull and inexpressive, with a few slight traces of make-up, probably applied in a hurry. Nothing in her appearance—her dress or expression, could make anyone suspect her tumultuous past. She was sitting quietly, almost resigned on the exam table as if she were alone, only with herself, like a forgotten old Greek statue, vandalized many times, still proud on her pedestal. When I examined the back of her thorax, I saw a large scar right under her shoulder blade.

"And this one?" I dared ask.

"The same knife. They had to operate on me. My lung collapsed and I bled a lot. I stayed in the hospital for three weeks."

"For God's sake, why did he do this to you?" I couldn't help asking.

"I don't know!" she repeated the words "passion" and "jealously" flatly, emptied of any emotional charge. She simply shrugged her shoulders.

When I checked her thyroid gland, I noticed a scar that went around her neck from one side to the other.

"Thyroid surgery?" I asked hesitantly, trying to hold on to a trace of professionalism.

"No. Same kitchen knife... A year after the breasts... he was obsessed with me, doctor. That's why I speak so slowly! He hit my vocal cords with the blade!"

Yes, she did speak a bit hoarsely, but that was not the problem. It was the empty and inexpressive tone in her voice when she talked about those horrible events, as if they hadn't really happened.

"The same man?" I asked.

"No. He was in jail. It was a friend of his whom I got involved with for a while. It happened while I was staying in the same place, the same singles' dorms!"

"For God's sake, what did they want from you?" I said automatically, sounding almost out of control. It was hard to believe that the woman who was sitting in front of me, shy, quiet, and resigned, carrying all those scars, could trigger such anger and fury. I tried to imagine her in her teen years, younger, thinner, and surely more joyful, in that damn industrial city, where she might have been pouring melted steel during the night shifts, or could have been one of the secretaries, one who placidly answered phone calls and made hot coffee for her boss. Then she added:

"Doctor, I try not to think about all this! Tough times! Too much vodka, jealousy, passion... Who knows?"

The nurse who was assisting me and who didn't understand Romanian, stared at us with her eyes wide open. I took a deep breath and tried to keep a neutral attitude. Only when I examined her genitals did I see the scars on her abdomen. Three of them. A large one above the umbilicus. She volunteered to tell me directly:

"The big one is also from Galati. The doctor thought I had a perforated ulcer. I knew the doctor well; we were involved for a few months…"

"With the scalpel?"

"Of course! With anesthesia, in the county hospital. I was in great pain, but they screwed it up. It wasn't a perforated ulcer. They cut me below also. Tubes for drainage, perfusions, another two weeks in the hospital. They removed a chunk of my intestine. The bottom one is from Brooklyn. They operated on me by mistake three years ago… a cyst had broken. I can't remember…"

I kept my composure and tried to examine her with a mind, emptied of the image of all her scars. Otherwise her genital exam was unremarkable. She quickly got off the table, but with some difficulty, slightly limping. That's when I saw a scar that went from her hip all the way down to her knee.

"What about your leg?" I asked terrified.

"Just a car accident… my new boyfriend! Open fracture. I have a metal rod in the femur. Sometimes he drinks, nerves, jealousy…"

I let her get dressed in silence and walked out completely baffled. In the waiting room I saw a tall muscular American man with his head completely shaved. He had an arrogant expression and threw me a nasty look while his feet involuntarily pounded the floor. He might have just been suffering from that new condition called "restless leg syndrome," which always sounded bizarre to me. Or he was just a nervous, jealous, passionate man? Who knows!

Miss M. came out from the exam room and whispered very slowly, in our native language:

"He's the guy from the accident… He feels sorry and now wants to marry me. I don't know what to say…"

They walked away quietly, holding hands like happy couples do.

This was a woman who'd instinctively learned how to handle the abuses of two different worlds. No therapist taught her how to heal or manage all the scars she was carrying. She seemed completely resigned. Next year she came back to my office pregnant. Showing her the fetus on the ultrasound screen, I made her smile for the first time. That baby was her miracle and everything went fine until she approached her due date and went into labor. The baby was pretty large and she was way passed 40. "Are going to cut me?" she asked me bluntly, trying to cope with the labor pains. Her question gave me goose bumps because I was seriously considering a cesarean delivery. I was thinking how I'd squeeze this new scar among all her old scars. At the end, I didn't have to do much because the baby's head rotated in the right position and she managed to push him out on her own.

LATE LOVE

LADY G WAS NEITHER eccentric nor obsessed by the myth of eternal youth. She seemed to be a very down to earth woman, one who accepted and even enjoyed menopause as a natural transition towards wisdom and serenity. She'd given birth naturally and raised two children who were now married, settled, and on their own. She hadn't had any kind of cosmetic surgery, or breast implants, nor did she have the immobile sphinx-like expression of those who abuse Botox, but she didn't hide her thick waist and wrinkles, only her walking was getting a little heavier.

I took care of her daughter's pregnancy, and Lady G was present for all the prenatal care sessions and was there when her first granddaughter was born. I figured out that Lady G was the one who had convinced her daughter to deliver by caesarian section. I personally considered that it would have been more appropriate to try natural birth, but in the end, Lady G persuaded her daughter to ask me for a surgical delivery. "Doctor, I don't want her to be like me," said Lady G a few times.

"What happened when you gave birth?" I asked her.

"Vaginal delivery. It's a risky business, doctor! At least in Romania back in those years. You worked there and know how it was..."

I didn't want to contradict her, because I'd been there in "those years." Lady G was present in the Operating Room, and with the first screams of the newborn, she seemed to be the happiest and most normal of all the world's grandmothers. At some point, enthused by the calm rhythm and ease of the operation, she asked me whether I did gynecological surgery, as well. When I told her I did, she said: "Perfect, doctor. I'll soon be your patient!"

I saw her again in the next few days because Lady G was always helping her daughter. She was constantly in the company of a young man, tall and handsome, who I believed to be the father of the newborn. I saw them in the hospital's corridors happily holding hands and told myself that she must have been a loving and caring mother-in-law. And she certainly was. Only that the baby's father was an officer in the U.S. Army and he was getting ready to be sent to Iraq. He showed up the day I released his wife. He seemed to be a typical American soldier, a Marine with shaved head, dressed in uniform. He gave me a military salute, thanked me for everything that I had done; moreover, when I asked him if he was happy to have a daughter, he responded with a military "Yes Sir!" that had a lot of heart in it.

"Fortunately, my mother-in-law will be here to help. She's great."

Lady G became my patient once her daughter's post-partum visits were done. In the beginning, as many other women, she felt embarrassed that she had to get undressed and expose herself naked in front of me. I tried to make her comfortable, and only after I fully examined her did she reveal the reason she was there:

"You asked me if I lose urine when I cough or sneeze. Yes, I have urine loss even when I laugh or run after the bus.

It's been happening for a while, but this is not what bothers me the most! The main problem is that it's too large!" There followed a short moment of silence, then she added: "Actually, it is him who complains of that..."

"Who complains?"

"You saw him when my daughter gave birth. He was there." There was another moment of silence that I didn't know how to fill, afraid not to mess things up. I still believed that the young man was her son or nephew.

"He keeps teasing me about this! Oh doctor, he read somewhere that nowadays there are vaginal procedures that can tailor our vaginas. He keeps saying that he loves me, but that it's too large... He thinks that's the reason we don't fit. You know what happens with age and vaginal deliveries, it gets wider. Sorry doc, I'm really embarrassed!"

How American I've become in these twenty years! I didn't ask any extra questions, as if I heard many such confessions, or as if I was used to be asked to perform a vaginoplasty every day. For a second, I tried to imagine what a Romanian doctor's reaction would have been, after being taken by surprise by such a request. In America, even our thoughts seem to have become politically correct, which is pretty scary. In the end, I don't believe it's always right to refrain from *expressing* your thoughts.

Lady G had an obvious genital prolapse, caused by the two difficult vaginal deliveries she had, and her bladder had dropped even lower. Both conditions should have been operated on to correct the problem. What hit me though was the motive for which she wanted to get on the operating table. By then, Lady G didn't say a word and was just looking down, somehow ashamed, like a woman who didn't know how to cope with a pitiful situation that came upon her by mistake.

All of a sudden, I felt that I was her accomplice, which seemed to ease the embarrassment between us.

As a gynecologist, it is quite often that I feel that I'm the accomplice to some patients, mainly when the patients go beyond a certain limit of confidentiality. Not necessarily when it's about a bodily condition, but mostly when it comes to the intimacy linked to that problem. Many young women who deliver children vaginally later develop a genital prolapse, which may be more or less symptomatic. A common problem is urinary incontinence, but most women want to have surgery because their vagina has become too large.

Not long before Lady G, I had a patient from Central America who didn't speak any English, yet we managed to communicate pretty well by using the Spanish I knew while she used body language. The main reason she wanted surgery was that her vagina made a certain unpleasant sound when she had sex. To convince me she tried to imitate that sound, as that sound would have been the main indication for surgery. I refused to operate on her because she was too young, didn't have any urinary incontinence, and the enlargement of her vagina wasn't so obvious. She confessed that she wanted surgery only to please her last lover who had complained a few times. In the end she went somewhere in the Dominican Republic to take care of the surgery. When she came back, she returned to me saying she didn't feel well. She had fever and pains because the vaginal wound had gotten infected. She had to be hospitalized and ended up with a vaginal stricture that was going to make her sex-life miserable for her entire life.

Lady G, who was far from her youthful days, told me: "I've been seen by a doctor in a private clinic, but I didn't like it. He said that he could make it like new for $6,000. Have you heard about this clinic?" She handed me a business card with the name of a clinic that I'd never heard of. "What do you think, doctor? Can you can help me?"

The truth was that Lady G had a real anatomical problem that only would have gotten worse with time. I explained to her in detail what the operation would entail and all the options, and of course, the risks. She asked me to schedule her for surgery as soon as possible. When she left, she asked me timidly how long the recovery would last.

"Between six and eight weeks. And no sex!"

She looked disturbed, seriously counting and thinking.

"God Almighty, that long… It's not about me, doctor! I'm thinking about him, poor man…"

The whole procedure turned out fine. In Romania in the old days, it was called the operation for "old perineal rupture" because the whole problem was caused by the laceration of the perineal muscles during vaginal deliveries. I don't know what they call it today, but back then it had a simple and generic diagnostic name, "rupture" deriving from a harsh and troubled history. In the States, besides the vaginal repair itself, meaning the tightening and reconstruction of the vaginal walls, we used to place a non-absorbing special sling under the urethra which would cure urinary loss. It is a relatively new technique and requires the use of certain special needles that must be introduced through the pelvis on a very precise trajectory, which go under the urethra and close to some major arteries. The complications can be disastrous if damage is done to blood vessels. This new method was introduced in the U.S. after it had been invented in Sweden and tested in Europe and Asia for many years.

This procedure has probably been abused, performed incompletely or incorrectly in some clinics, often executed just for cosmetic reasons for patients who were convinced that they would walk away with a vagina "good as new." There are similar procedures pompously called "vaginal rejuvenation," not standardized or approved by the American College of Gynecology, performed by licensed doctors in exchange for large sums of money. These are surgical procedures balanced between science and deception.

Years ago a private patient convinced me to operate on her because she complained that her labia was too large. I tried to tell her that many women have large labias and that wasn't a good enough reason to operate. In the end, she managed to convince me to take her into the Operating Room, because her labia became really inflamed and swollen when she worked out in the gym. I asked for advice and our Chief surgeon showed me that there is a standard procedure called a labial reduction that has a code that is paid by insurance. My patient was asked to pay $4,000 at a private clinic that specialized in "vaginal rejuvenations." I would have felt ridiculous to get her in the OR when there wasn't a clear indication for surgery.

The operation for a labia reduction is a very simple one. As with all cases of vaginoplasty, one has to trim tissues with care, following a simple principle that from much you get to less, but from less you can't get much more. In the end, I felt that somehow I'd been cheated. Not because the insurance wouldn't reimburse me, but only because the patient told me later that this was just the beginning of a process of beautification and reshaping of her body. She was still a young and beautiful woman with a nice harmonious body.

I had assisted one of her three deliveries. She was thirty-eight but looked much younger. The kids were already grown up, and her seventeen-year-old daughter had already made her a grandma. I thought she should have done nothing more but enjoy the life that seemed to boil inside her as wildly as soup in a pot that had blown its lid off.

"Thank you, doctor! Wait and see what's next! As soon as my labia heals, I'll put a ring through my clitoris, possibly a small tattoo around it too. I haven't decided yet. My cousin did something similar and it looks fantastic. This is just the beginning, doctor! In three months I'll be in the Dominican Republic where I'll fix my breasts with silicon and thicken my lips. At least I don't have wrinkles, thank God, but these guys also do body sculpting. They'll take fat from my back and belly and put it on my buttocks to make it round and hard as an apple. Then the birth marks, I'll..."

"You have no birth marks and your butt is OK," I screamed almost desperate, at the edge of making an inappropriate comment.

The patient was not at all impressed by my intervention and kept going. "Doctor, doctor! You're a man. You don't understand! Beyond my age, the competition gets intense! I have four younger cousins ready to steal my new boyfriend!"

I remained speechless.

I remembered an article published in *The Wall Street Journal* covering this new trend in personal beautification. It was about a private clinic located in Queens, New York, run by a Cuban woman who wasn't a licensed doctor. Amongst other things, they were performing a so called hymeno-plasty, meaning the rebuilding of the hymen, to restore the lost virginity, all for $5,000. It was advertised as a very simple "operation," that could be done in an office under local anesthesia, if indicated, for God's sake! They were also doing some more sophisticated procedures which all belonged to the same named "vaginal rejuvenation" group of procedures. It was this very clinic that offered to perform the operation for Lady G. The whole story stirred my curiosity.

The next day I was at the doors of that clinic which I found with some difficulty because the entrance seemed to be the ground door to an average two story duplex apartment, typical for Ridgewood, Queens. The lady who opened the door was the owner and manager of the clinic. She also ran a local Spanish publication that advertised beautification and "vaginal rejuvenation" for women. She told me that they were interested in hiring gynecologists with experience in the field. They were doing Botox treatments also, as well as laser removal for unwanted hair, and other simple procedures that I could easily learn. All done for cash. She asked me if I knew how to do the new sling procedure and suddenly became more interested in my skills. As we were talking, she became more relaxed, observing that I was a foreigner myself with an accent and the desire for free enterprise. She decided to show me the rest of the clinic, which proved to be larger than I expected. We came out of the small room, and I was surprised when she walked me through five or six Operating Rooms which were all hidden inside the apparently small and modest building. A few doctors were at work along with nurses, anesthesiologists, and assistants dressed in scrubs.

It seemed to be a small ambulatory surgical clinic, only one would not have expected to see Operating Rooms crammed into a small space next to pizzerias, hair salons and Chinese fast food eateries. I guessed the clinic must have had all the permits it needed; otherwise the police would have closed it a long time ago. The reality is that since I've been in New York, I've seen many businesses and companies operating on the edge, with law firms on the watch at every corner.

For procedures that were either not allowed, or too expensive in the U.S., the owner of the surgical clinic arranged transportation and accommodation in Santo Domingo, plus a week of recovery time on the beach, all for less than a third of American prices. In the end, she told me frankly that it was a pity for a gynecologist with my experience to waste his time working hard in a first line hospital in Queens for such little money. "What do you think, doc? Are you going to work for us?"

I left the place sick and tired, thinking of the difficult night of 'on-call's' when we work for twenty-four hours for less than doctors got paid in that clinic for one simple procedure!

I made a little mistake with Lady G. I forgot to ask her how big her lover's penis was. When I started performing this type of surgery in Romania, my mentors use to tell us that it was best to ask the patient about the size of her husband's penis in order to "tailor" the restored vagina. But in the States I did not ask this question, as it could have been perceived as too invasive. There is a real risk to tighten a vagina too much and create strictures that would have made intercourse much more painful.

Everybody knows that the size of the penis varies a great deal between men, and it's good to have some idea before the operation. The procedure is made in two stages; the first stage is for the repair of the anterior wall of the vagina (and the sling is applied under the urethra) and a different sling is made for the posterior wall, which may be avoided if the vagina becomes too narrow. Lady G was very happy with the immediate result of the operation because she miraculously stopped losing urine. But three months later, she wasn't happy any longer.

"Doctor, it's still too large. He keeps complaining."

I examined her carefully, and everything seemed just right. I asked her to wait a few more months hoping that things would settle in more smoothly. After six months, she came back with tears in her eyes. She was waiting with her lover, the same young guy who had a frustrated look on his face. He looked at me disappointed, even disrespectful, and I had a hint something wasn't right. I examined Lady G and tried to convince her that everything looked fine.

"No, doctor, it's not fine. You said that you could tighten it a bit more in the "posterior," and that's why I'm here. I'm begging you to do the second step as well."

I could have refused but her knees and her elbows convinced me. She had obvious bruises on both, as kids have when they fall and scratch themselves.

"Did you fall?" I dared ask her and saw her blush for the first time.

"I didn't fall. I tried to satisfy him the way I can… It's not easy at my age, trust me." That was what convinced me. I immediately scheduled her to correct the back part of her vaginal wall. The operation went well, but I had slight worries that I might have overdone the tightening.

Lady G went home the same day and for a while I forgot about her. She came back in three months and looked sadder than ever. She was there in the waiting room with her lover and both gave me angry looks. What I appreciated about Lady G was that the she would always step alone into the consultation room. We both felt that it would have been too much to have him there as well.

"How is it?" I asked anxiously. I was scared that now it had become too narrow, which was worse than too large.

"Bad." She put it simply. I quietly examined her. Everything was well healed. Then I saw her knees. She had fresh bruises on both, like second degree burns on which she must have applied skin lotion.

"Too tight?" I asked her terrified.

"Not at all. He says it's still too large! Did you see my knees? I try all kind of positions, only to please him. Even my back hurts. I'm desperate!"

I finally asked her what I should have asked her a long time ago: "Excuse me, but how big is his penis?"

"It's small. Very small! Do you want me to draw it?"

I nodded, and she picked up one of my prescription pads, grabbed my pen, which I was nervously playing with, and in a few strokes, drafted a very small sketch.

"Do you understand me now?"

I knew there was nothing else I could do.

INHERITANCE

"WHEN DO YOU THINK this 'miracle' will happen? I can't wait any longer!" she asked me anxiously, taking a glimpse at her wrist watch, as if she could move time forward when we all wanted to move it back. She was a beautiful middle aged woman, who looked at least ten years younger: that is, I was willing to dismiss a few details that usually won't lie and cannot be changed by any aesthetic surgery. Like the real age of our hands. When it comes to men, the hands get wider with age. In the last twenty years, my own hands have gotten bigger, so in the Operating Room I need size eight gloves, instead of size seven which used to fit me when I started.

"I don't know when it will happen," I answered. "Nobody can predict something like that. It's an issue of inheritance."

"Inheritance? From whom?"

"From your mother! Each woman gets a few hundred thousand follicles before she's even born: between two hundred and six hundred thousand."

"Follicles?" She looked at me pleasantly surprised, as if I was talking about a precious inheritance, some diamonds or rubies she wasn't aware of.

"Yes, the follicles in your ovaries... You're born with a limited number: you 'inherit' them from the time you are six months-old in your mother's womb."

"So, when we're born, the biological clock is already set in our ovaries?" She looked at me scared, as if she was peering at a huge pendulum on the wall from where a cuckoo might un-expectantly pop out saying: cuckoo, it's menopause time!

"Something like that... But why are you so anxiously waiting for it?"

"I'm fed up with all these cycles, the heavy bleeding, the clots, the premenstrual symptoms, the gloom and crying that comes out of the blue. Then, there is my fibroid uterus which you say is getting bigger! I want my body to quiet down and steady my hormones, like you, men, have."

"Hmm." I wanted to say something but I just mumbled.

I had known Susan for many years. I knew her husband, her two daughters—the younger one being delivered by me years ago under rather dramatic circumstances. She had been pregnant, coming back from Europe, and when flying over Greenland her labor pains started way before term. When the plane landed at JFK, she was bleeding badly. The ambulance picked her up from the runway and brought her to Jamaica Hospital, where I was 'on-call.'

We became family friends, kept in touch over the years, and she'd contact me often for medical advice even when the issue was not a gynecological one. We would see each other in Manhattan in some art circles where I was known mostly as a writer. She would introduce me protectively while holding my arm: "He's my gynecologist from Queens! I would not trade him for anything in the world." When she said "Queens" she would use a peculiar tone as she was talking about the moon, or about a strange invisible planet, a place where the ones who live in Manhattan—definitely a different planet—happen to pass through only when going to the New York airports.

Overall, we all live on a thrilling planet, that of New York City, where nobody knows who's more Martian than the other. My doctor-patient relationship with Susan had always been a special one, creative, never monotonous, based on mutual trust and respect, peppered with a little Eastern European humor from my side and some nicely veiled tragic-comic and brilliant refinements from her side.

In the last few years I've managed to convince Susan that she didn't need any procedure for her fibroid uterus. Nothing "robotic" like embolization, or aesthetic, or "using lasers," because those small fibroids didn't bother her and were quietly waiting in their place for menopause to come. Then they would get smaller and eventually be forgotten. And menopause, dear Susan, would come when it was due to come. Why should we rush it? Most women don't want to go through menopause, but Susan, a woman made to challenge the passage of time, was waiting for it with a strange impatience as if it would be some sort of cure for her problems, even though she wasn't sure what they were... I think that was the only aspect of her life which didn't fit with who she really was. Maybe she was just playing a subconscious game, being afraid of menopause. Once she asked me plainly, like a spoiled child would ask about a contagious disease: "And when it comes, how long will it last?"

How could I answer such a question? Would it be enough to say that menopause is a natural and permanent state, neither an illness, nor a condition, nor a syndrome to suffer through? Many women enter this phase with a simple shrug and a smile on their lips. But seen as a room with only an entrance door, menopause might not be comforting at all, just a life stage, which women are not in a rush to live through. Some suffer a lot, and beside hot flushes, they complain that they can't recognize their own bodies, minds or basic dreams anymore. It's a very personal passage, different from woman to woman. I am often asked to give advice, mainly to patients I have known for many years. I might have delivered their children, seen how they changed over the years, or witnessed their first wrinkles. Some are close to my own age and expect more empathy, more solutions on my part.

Susan was definitely a different case, extreme in her way. When she asked me how long menopause would last, she stumped me. I mumbled only that it would come and go as all things do in life, which didn't satisfy her at all.

She somehow reminded me of a strange interview I had seen on Romanian TV years ago. A biased reporter had randomly quizzed hundreds of women and men in the streets about what they thought about menopause. The answers were stupefying because many women didn't know what menopause was, and not wanting to look ignorant, came out with incredible answers. One said that when menopause comes, she would quietly sit on a bench in the factory's park, watching the birds while eating her sandwich. Another one, when asked whether men should also go through menopause, said "sure, poor men deserve menopause because they work hard enough." So this life phase was mostly viewed as a well-deserved pause for everybody!

"Eh, you're a man. What do you care!" Susan told me. "You don't go through what we go through every month! How old are you? Don't tell me we're are the same age," she added, not expecting any answer.

I tried to picture Susan and myself in the same room ten or twenty years later, a bit older, talking about menopause and andropause, because men don't stay unchanged with age either. In the 1990's my hospital sent me to open a new clinic in The Rockaways, Brooklyn, in an Italian neighborhood with second and third generation immigrants. There, Rici Sorento Jr., an over eighty-year-old gynecologist, was still seeing patients because that was his profession and business and he didn't want to suddenly quit. He was smoking in his office, a habit that today is banned even in New York parks. I could hear him from the next room coughing and talking to his patients, women almost his age whose children and grandchildren he'd delivered—women who now consoled him about his bad health and the cough he couldn't control. Before leaving, they used to hug, encourage and tenderly comfort him. "Don't worry Rici, everything will be alright, just take it easy with your smoking."

When Susan asked me about menopause, she probably just needed some reassurance, and I should have done better with that. Sometimes it is so easy to give people hope. I am good at that, but I told myself that menopause isn't an incurable disease, and Susan seemed to be in perfect control of her being. I knew that she saw a few other doctors in Manhattan because once in a while she would call and ask me peculiar questions, like was it possible to delay menopause, or make it come early.

I didn't see her for the next two years, nor did I meet her at any literary event in the city. One afternoon I found her waiting in my office. She showed up before I started seeing patients, and I quickly understood that something unusual had happened. She had a troubled look, red eyes, filed with wrath. I don't know why, but she made me feel somehow guilty, as men sometimes feel for no reason.

"Susan, so nice to see you..."

"Yeah, sure! Come on! Be honest: you haven't thought a minute of me all these years."

She stunned me, and for a few seconds I quickly recalled everything I'd remembered about her, but in front of me stood a different woman.

"Oh, forgive me!" she said, her voice trembling and her eyes tearing-up.

A woman who cries can have a great impact on me.

"What happened to you?" I asked with in a professional voice.

"I really don't know. For more than a year I feel that I haven't been myself."

"Did you go through menopause?"

"No way! I have my period every month, like clockwork! It's about my mind and my body.... They're not mine anymore. It's a long story. Do you want to know how it started?"

"Yes," I nodded; I wanted to hear her story to understand what had changed in her.

"A year ago, Stanley, my husband whom you know well, organized a surprise birthday party for me. I tortured Stanley with my mood swings, and the poor man only wanted to make me happy. Thank God he forgot to invite you. As it goes, our house was full of friends, lights off, and me coming straight from the gym sweating like a horse all pumped with adrenaline. Suspecting nothing. I walk in, and everybody shouts: "Surprise!" The lights went on. There was confetti and trumpets. Honestly, after all the crap Stanley got from me, that was impressive. I smiled crookedly, had one or two drinks with them, exchanged a few meaningless words and then, out of the blue, I went berserk and flipped out. Yep, it was pretty ugly!"

Susan started to sob again.

"Guess what I did next?"

I just shrugged.

"I grabbed a huge cake knife, and, ranting badly, I asked them all to leave. Immediately! It was like I was possessed. The people got scared and ran out. Stanley went to the bedroom, shoved his head in the pillows and began to cry, just as I'm crying now. Subdued and hopeless! Then I felt such pity for Stanley and tried to comfort him, but he was so scared that he screamed at the top of his lungs. I realized that I was still holding the knife in my hand. I threw it through the window, knelt in from of him, begged for forgiveness, telling him that I didn't know what I was doing anymore. Then I heard the knife hit the sidewalk. You know that we live on the fortieth floor? Thank God nobody got hurt! May I continue?" she asked, with doubt in her voice. I nodded.

"I saw a few doctors, but they didn't help. Stanley said, 'try your Queens gynecologist also.'" She looked at me to see how I'd react, or perhaps to just remember how a Queens gynecologist looked. Then she continued: "What else do you think I did that night? I got on top of Stanley in bed and I would say that I raped him. Do you think a woman can rape a man? What do you think about that? Are you called in to the Emergency Room for rape cases?"

"Yes, we are!" I said. "Last week they called me for a six-year-old girl. It's terrible. I don't even want to think of it."

"But I don't believe you've ever been called for a raped man," Susan went on, still crying softly. "Poor Stanley! He still loves me. A woman can't rape a man if he doesn't love her. What do you think? That night, when I climaxed, I screamed so loudly that our neighbors banged on the walls. They thought I'd killed him. I buried my nails in his back and ripped his skin from top to bottom. I'm not lying. I had his flesh under my fingernails. He bled, went to the ER, and needed bandages for a week."

Instinctively, I grimaced, which she didn't miss. She stopped her narrative for a second, just to give me a chance to recover. In the meantime, the door opened and my assistant stuck her head in to see if everything was OK and to tell me discreetly that there were patients waiting for me.

"This was just the beginning," she added gravely. "I wonder why Stanley kept living under the same roof with me. I went to a psychiatrist who gave me strong sedatives that made me wobbly in the house, jogging through Central Park in zigzags, and I got lost a couple of times. Then came the anti-depressants. I was told that I'm bipolar and switched to lithium, as if I was a broken battery. The endocrinologist told me that I have hyperthyroidism, although the blood tests were fine. Then I went through homeopathy, psychotherapy, acupuncture, and hypnosis. You want more? I did meditation with a guru. I believe we live in a city with the most psychotherapists and gurus per capita in the entire world! There are as many as you need, from everywhere: India, Tibet, the Philippines, even from your country. You know that I stumbled on one from Transylvania, who said that he has magnetic powers that would help me get into an unbelievable deep trance. Bullshit! I went somewhere upstate and stayed in isolation for a month, in an expensive camp, eating only salads, repeating all kinds of mantras, learning to look at my inside until I got fed up with myself. This is about the phase I am in right now. I have no clue what else to do. I'm scared! Stanley wants to run away to Australia… Help me! Maybe you have an idea!"

How could I help her? I was speechless and clueless as to what to do, so I just performed a routine check up on her. She'd lost weight, looked tired and acted neurotic, otherwise I couldn't find anything abnormal. I convinced her to have a mammography and wanted to get some blood for routine tests. She rolled up her sleeve. I wrapped her arm with a rubber tube to find some veins, even if that wasn't necessary, because she had muscular arms and the veins were visible.

"Why do you want to get my blood?" She asked suspiciously.

"To see if you're getting close to menopause. Plus, the thyroid..."

Susan got rid of the rubber tube and quickly pulled her sleeve down, somehow angry.

"There is no need! I've been tested not long ago by my Primary Care doctor. I told you that I have my menses monthly!"

She left me perplexed, standing with the needle in my hand, staring at me as if I were a vampire from one of the stupid Dracula movies from Transylvania, my homeland. Each time I've been asked about this American cliché, I try to resist and ridicule it as much as I can. In Germany, Romanian immigrants would say that they come from "Siebenburgen", and not from Transylvania, which sounds better in Europe. But when you say Transylvania in the States, you can see an immediate queer smile, not necessarily malicious, and the name Dracula is quickly mentioned.

Susan's visit came to a sudden end, but she still asked me: "Didn't you say that menses stop when we reach menopause?"

"That's right! Are you sure you aren't taking other drugs? Chinese ginseng or some hormones?"

A long pause followed. No Answer. Susan seemed to be playing a role that she acted with difficulty. She left, leaving behind a mixed taste of trouble and sadness, unevenly sprinkled with a fury hard to control. Before she departed, she ventured to ask:

"Can you recommend something for my libido? The truth is, it's dying… Something like your damn Viagra! Wouldn't it be unjust not to have something for women!"

I told her that the only hormone that would stimulate the libido, including in women, is testosterone. Sadly, during those days there was no drug with testosterone in American pharmacies. I still wonder why not. Not for women, nor for men, as if testosterone were an illegal and dangerous drug, not at all like amphetamines, sleeping pills, pain killers with morphine, barbiturates, tranquilizers, which kill thousands of young people each night in their sleep. Addicts on prescriptions created by doctors. Drugs given away with great ease, tragedies with no end in sight. We notice this only when a celebrity dies and two or three pill vials are shown on the nightstand with the doctor's name on them. In the end, nobody is at fault. The profit for a product like testosterone must be very small, otherwise I can't explain why there is no testosterone cream on the market! So, when Susan asked me to give her something for her libido, all I could do was shrug my shoulders.

After she left I called her family doctor whom I knew well and asked to have her tests sent to me; her menopause tests had been ordered only to be cancelled later on. Why hadn't Susan want me or her to know whether she'd reached menopause? Why was she so scared?

I remembered that one time when we'd met at a literary event in Manhattan, we got to talk about American and Eastern European myths. Then I told her about a fairytale called *Youth Without Old Age and Life Without Death*, which we learned in school, a kind of folk-legend which had been transmitted orally through the ages. The story resonated with Susan, and she asked me if there was any English translation, which made me smile, but she was put off by my reaction.

"You Eastern Europeans have a very strange attitude when it comes to these 'existential issues.'"

"Are you talking about old age and death?" I asked her, maybe in too loud of a voice.

"Not so loud, please! I am not deaf. These words must be uttered with utmost care and as seldom as we can!"

I looked at her carefully and realized that Susan was not a typical American woman, if something like that even exits. She was somehow lacking the firm-sturdy Anglo-Saxon structure that does not shudder in the face of strong words and facts. I thought that our myths about utopic youth without old age and life without death would better fit here in New York, and America at large, where people try to avoid these topics by ignoring them.

I hadn't seen or heard from Susan for a few good months. Then, late one night when I was deeply asleep, my cell went off, repeating a part of a Louis Armstrong song. I thought a pregnant woman was ready to deliver. When I answered the phone, Susan went straight to the point:

"I managed to find gel with testosterone from Canada. I need advice, right away! Can I use it with contraceptive pills?"

"Why do you take birth control pills?" I mumbled somewhat upset.

"At first, I didn't want to get pregnant. Besides, I feel much better when I'm on them. The problem is that Stanley is about to leave me! Please!"

"Who prescribed you contraceptives?"

"Nobody. They are leftovers from my daughter. Listen doc, that's not why I called you! Can I use the testosterone cream? Excellent! So just spread a bit of gel on the forearm? Thank you, darling. Have a good night!"

Six months later we came face to face during the intermission of a ballet at Lincoln Center. She'd gained a little weight and looked very well. Her eyes had the live expression I remembered, ironic, smart, and cunning, although it was clear that some plastic surgery had been done in the meantime. She was with Stanley, but he looked much older, even though it was obvious that he was dying his hair. We were soon joined by a tall and svelte lady who returned smiling from the bar with a glass of champagne in hand.

"She's my mother!" Susan made the introductions.

They did look very much alike and both seemed to have an uncertain age, frozen in time.

"I hope to be like her," Susan added. "You said that it's a matter of 'inheritance!'"

We shook hands warmly and exchanged a few enthusiastic words about the ballet we'd just seen. It was Ravel's Bolero: a tall and supple flamenco ballerina danced fabulously, sensuous and dramatic, on that crescendo rhythm, in front of a group of male dancers who hypnotically surrounded her from all sides. Before we went back to our seats I said discreetly:

"You look good, just as I've known you for all these years!"

"Merci, darling! I am better than ever, even though I reached, menopause!" She pronounced the last word discreetly into my ear as if it was a secret that only the two of us knew.

"Why don't you translate that myth of yours? The one about old age and life without death. Should be a great success here..." Susan told me.

I followed her with my eyes. She seemed to be reborn. She had the walk of a young woman, up right, with tight and healthy skin, in spite of a light shadow above her upper lip, which only a specialist might have understood.

"V" FOR VACCINE

AS I GOT TO THE HOSPITAL, the department secretary called out to me. She was a nice friendly woman who in the same courtly professional voice would let you know that you forgot to punch in for the day, the Christmas party had just been scheduled, or perhaps that you've been temporarily suspended. I'm sure that she would announce the end of the world in the same warm polite voice. That Friday, she told me I was the only doctor in our department who hadn't gotten his flu shot and it was the last day to do so. Otherwise, starting the next Monday, I wouldn't be able to enter the hospital. To be more specific, when trying to sign in by placing my finger on the diabolic electronic gadget that reads our fingerprints, I wouldn't be allowed in my hospital anymore. All its electronic doors, which I've entered freely for the last 20 years, would be shut to me. We're talking here about a New York City hospital, not a nuclear power plant or a National Security Administration facility.

On my lunch break I headed straight to our clinic used for hospital personnel. Here, in the United States, every hospital has its own medical office for its employees which is run like an odd Ministry of Interior of a small country. I had to complete three long forms calling for lots of personal data, which I then handed to the nurse. Ten minutes passed while I tried to decide which shoulder to be pricked; then she told me that it was better to come back after lunch since the doctor was out.

I got out fast, determined to forget the whole vaccine process and go bravely through that winter's perils using my own immune system just as the good Lord made it. Up until a year ago, we were vaccinated on the spot, wherever they could get hold of us. You didn't even have time to react. Every corridor had two efficient nurses stationed at a desk. You passed by them on the way to attend to something or other, and they would stop you: "Did you get your flu shot, dear? You didn't? Come here, please." While one wrote your name down in a register, the other would roll up your sleeve, and before you could react, she'd professionally stick the needle in your shoulder.

You could even skip the flu shot altogether, and some did just that. The number of those who skipped the flu shot grew in direct proportion to the number of conspiracy theories over the years. Two or three years ago there was talk that the government wanted to implant a small chip under our skin and use it to track us for the rest of our lives. Even with that risk, I got the flu shot almost every year. Besides, I wanted to be tracked, and this is not because of some strange syndrome I suffer from. I travel abroad a lot and hope that I will be more easily found if I get lost. Sometimes I just forgot to get vaccinated which in a way proved not only that we're not tracked, but that the government really doesn't give a damn.

As I left the clinic I bumped into one of our administrative chiefs, a tough, very powerful person, who makes everyone nervous, because every dollar that reaches us passes through his fingers. "Doctor Sangerhozan" he called loudly—sometimes the mispronunciation of my name in English gives me goose bumps—"you didn't get your vaccine! This is the last day!"

I remained calm and tried to defend myself, saying that I was just coming from the medical office.

"But you didn't get it yet, did you?"

With this he upset me, just like in my childhood when I was caught lying. How did he know that the nurse didn't prick me with the needle yet? I thought they must have a new kind of communication system that I was not aware of.

"How do you know that?" I asked. After all, I am one of the veterans of this hospital.

"Because you don't have the "V" sticker on your badge." He showed me his that, indeed, sported a big red V sticker.

"V for victory?" I asked trying to make a joke.

"V for vaccine," he replied bluntly. I didn't have a ready comeback. *The Vagina Monologues*, the old Broadway show came to mind, the play where one of the actors said "V" is for vagina.

I went to the hospital cafeteria to have lunch where I quickly fixed myself a large salad with nuts that made me healthier just by looking at them. I glanced around for somewhere to sit and finally found a place next to two anesthesiologists chatting with some nurses. One of them wore a face mask, and only then did I realize that many hospital workers were wearing similar face masks. The masks were the same as the kind we use in the OR. I suddenly felt strange and out of place. I had just returned from vacation and felt that perhaps an ugly flu epidemic may be hovering around, and there I was, walking unprotected among sick people. A woman next to me could barely feed herself. She lifted her mask just a bit, enough to be able to put some food in her mouth. I felt sorry for her, but I thought that she might just be a highly civic-minded person who didn't want to share her viruses with the rest of the hospital.

"Did you catch a cold? Why are you wearing a mask?" I asked her sympathetically.

"I'm not sick at all. I refused the flu shot, and now we must wear a mask."

"For how long?" I asked.

"No clue" she shrugged. "Maybe for the whole winter. They'll let us know when we can take it off."

Then she looked at my badge and said: "You should wear one too. You don't have the *V*... If you want one, I have a new one in my pocket."

I refused her offer and tried to swallow the rest of my salad.

Our cafeteria looked like a strange and freakish masked ball. I remembered Varanasi, India where many pilgrims wore masks because of the stench coming from the sewers, from the sacred cows that shat all over the place, and from the sick waiting patiently to die and be cremated on the Ganges. They hoped that their souls would go straight to heaven without any troublesome reincarnations. I have seen people wearing masks in China because of pollution, or in Thailand during the Chicken Flu epidemic. There, the masks seemed normal, protective, but not in our cafeteria where the wearers looked like scared tourists afraid to breathe any kind of air. I've seen Japanese tourists wearing these masks the world over, even in the Grand Canyon and the Peruvian Andes where one finds the world's cleanest air. One can't say who protects whom from what.

I decided to go back to our clinic where Dr. Patrick was waiting. I knew him well, a Pole with an Eastern European history similar to mine and whose last name I could never pronounce. He too cannot pronounce my name. For years during the '90s we worked together in a Brooklyn clinic. Every morning and every lunch break we talked about stocks and bonds. This was the time when Wall Street was sky-high and almost all Americans believed they would soon get rich and live like kings. We were both "day trading," naively making investments hoping to quickly become millionaires. Back then we lost lots of money that we still do not talk about to this day. There was a podiatrist that gave us prescient investment tips and a psychiatrist so detached from reality that he came to work in sandals even in the winter. Today the psychiatrist wears shoes, we recouped our losses, our children are grown, and when we meet, we talk about the countries we've escaped from. Eight or nine years ago, Patrick was still considering going back to Poland; today he doesn't want to even mention it.

We forgot about the vaccine and started talking about the general state of Europe, particularly the eastern region. Patrick made me feel good, as he always does, telling me that life in Poland wasn't much better than life in Romania. The current number one issue facing the nation we now live in is Obama-care. We both jumped on the subject and he agreed right away that I was at an advantage, being older and closer to retirement age. Patrick is more radical and pessimistic than I am because, "look, we all go together when we go, in this new homeland of ours."

I shook his hand and headed to the door, but he stopped me: "You forgot the vaccine!"

"What if I don't get it?"

"Hmmm! Then you have to wear a mask, but not any mask! Because you have a beard, a normal mask won't fit, so we have to order you a special one, bigger and more uncomfortable. That's only if you don't want to shave your beard...!"

Then he took the syringe out from the drawer and told me with a straight face: "You'd better pull up your sleeve. They're not kidding." He stabbed me with a special syringe that had lots of small needles which were painful. I rushed out the door again, but he called me back:

"You forgot the most important thing...," he said, and then he stuck the "V" on my ID badge, which would publicly prove my immunity and my good faith.

"V for vaccine, not for victory..." I mumbled. "V for vulnerability or for whatever you want..." We said goodbye in good spirits, with me finally vaccinated. When I got to the elevator I saw a nurse looking at my ID strangely, and I saw in the mirror that by mistake the sticker had been placed upside down. I left it that way to see what would happen.

In the old days, in the Romania of my childhood, vaccines came one after another because there were many infectious diseases that needed to be eradicated. No one objected to vaccinations. There weren't any conspiracy theories, because conspiracy theories had already been used with great success. For example, we had absolutely no idea that we kowtowed to Stalin, along with all of Eastern Europe. Our people were still naively waiting for the Americans to come. How could we know that at Yalta in 1945, on a cold winter day, Roosevelt, Stalin and Churchill redrew the map of Europe on a paper napkin that just happened to be on the table? The napkin was then used by one of them to blow his nose, without erasing the borders which held us prisoners for fifty years.

The first vaccines arrived in the '50s and '60s from the USSR. They were received with great enthusiasm by Romanians who wanted to get in line with the rest of the world. They didn't have a clue that in the process they would be massively infected with hepatitis B and C. This was not the Communist Party wanting to exterminate us, but simply negligence from not sterilizing the needles. Nobody bothered with such a small detail in a world so complicated and ruthless.

The first polio and chickenpox vaccines, of good quality otherwise, were used in the classrooms for "special" children, the offspring of the Communist nomenclature. Although the regime recommended careful sterilization, those nurses used, in a very democratic way, the same needle for everybody. Thus, over 30 children of ministers and state secretaries, from only one classroom, got infected with hepatitis C. Only three of them are still alive today, and I know this story from a good friend who was one of them and who lives and gets treatment in New York.

Recently, I delivered a young Romanian's firstborn. She was a woman infected with hepatitis C transmitted from her mother. When she was a child, her neighbor, who was a nurse and a good friend, would come by every autumn and inject the entire household with *Polidin,* an immune system stimulant. First she injected the mother to give the kids some courage; then she infected the rest of the family. The whole family got hepatitis C because their mother had contracted it from a blood transfusion in the hospital.

When I was in elementary school, they came to vaccinate us without notice. The teacher locked the door so we couldn't escape. Some children were crying, some tried to jump out the window, others had to be restrained. I would masochistically roll up my sleeve and always be the first to step up just to get away from all that craziness. Sometimes your premonition gives you the best advice. Those vaccines were a true delayed Russian Roulette which we played unknowingly. No one had an inkling what lay hidden in that casserole with those eternally re-sterilized needles. It was a lottery between life and death.

When I got to my hospital on Monday, every door had a security guard posted in front. We have a serious, very visible security service, a couple dozen sturdy men in uniform, about the same security force that a medium-size European city might have. They were checking our "V" on ID badges. My upside down "V" sticker didn't cause me any trouble. I believe that they were not as scared by the flu epidemic as they were by an audit by the State Department of Health. Recent regulations called for every person found unvaccinated or not wearing a mask, to be fined thousands of dollars, which would be paid directly from the hospital coffers. So the number of masked people had increased, and now we recognized each other with some difficulty.

AN EMERGENCY

SHE LOOKED PAPER-WHITE because she'd lost too much blood. More than she was eager to admit. She was that kind of woman who would describe any physical suffering as being far below its actual level. She'd bled gradually over a few weeks, and her young body had had time to adjust. If all of a sudden somebody got such a serious case of anemia, that person would have passed out right away.

She tried to convince me that she was well, not bothered by her pale skin, her dizziness, or even that once she had passed out in the street. Truth is that she looked well. As pale as she was, she resembled a saint, painted on an old byzantine church, only that we were in my gynecological office, and her blood results showed that she had severe anemia that should be treated as soon as possible. She shrugged her shoulders, as if she didn't care about her decreased hemoglobin level or even that she could drop dead or have a stroke. She needed a blood transfusion, and her bleeding could have been stopped in the Operating Room with a simple procedure. At the beginning, she didn't agree with any of these options and said that she would just take more iron and eat better food. I tried to convince her by using my model of a broken bucket—a mental representation of a vessel which loses water through its holes. Instead of fixing it, we kept pouring water in. It didn't work, and she didn't like the idea that I called her case "an emergency." From her reaction, I figured that I wouldn't come to an easy agreement with her. Another tough Eastern European woman completely taken with her job, family and life in New York City. The word "tough" should be pronounced with some kindness and graciousness, because although they look fragile, these women are strong enough to carry oversized burdens on their shoulders. They'd see a doctor only when they couldn't take it anymore; then they'd regret it because the doctor would tell them things they didn't want to hear. Some can live in complete denial of their own body as if they existed outside its reality. I didn't know much about my patient, but I guessed that she had a complicated life story, as most immigrants have. They just need some comfort and trust in conversation to open up and start telling their stories. I wished I had more time to listen to them to the end. Sometimes I think that their physical sufferings might be related to the complicated stories they carry.

Since I was 'on-call' in the hospital the next day, in the end, I convinced her to come to the E.R. I had to stop her bleeding and give her a blood transfusion in order for her to be removed from the category of "saints" with risks. She didn't like it, but the next day she came to the E.R. and quickly consented to go into the O.R. for a uterine curettage. When I told her that later she might need a hysterectomy she again shrugged her shoulders and said that she would never have that done. She had a small fibroid uterus that could grow worse over time. She refused the blood transfusion but agreed to the procedure, and when I tried to explain the risks, she stopped me. "Please, doctor. I don't need to hear about all these horrors. I trust you."

Based on this trust, we went into the O.R. and I did the procedure which took ten minutes and stopped the bleeding right away.

"Who's going to take you home?" I asked when she woke up from anesthesia. The hospital won't let you leave by yourself. She gave me a phone number, and the voice who answered the call was that of a man who seemed sleepy or perhaps drunk. He just hung up on me.

"Was that your husband?" I asked.

"No. It's my son. I'll find somebody else..."

I didn't see her again for almost a year. The pathology result was benign. My secretary called her a few times; then I forgot about her, until one day she came back to my office with a strange expression on her face, looking like a different person. She had lost a lot of weight, wasn't pale anymore, and didn't look at all like a byzantine saint, or any kind of saint because they don't cry and don't have red eyes.

"How are you doing?" I asked somehow intimidated. "Did you start bleeding again?"

"Not at all. But now I want to have surgery. As soon as possible. You said something about having a hysterectomy, right?"

"Why do you want surgery now? You have a small fibroma and just said that you feel well."

"I want it for different reasons. Can you schedule me for next week? The sooner the better."

I couldn't refrain from asking myself why she was in such a hurry to get rid of her uterus. Women don't easily accept this procedure, even when they really need it. A hysterectomy was, and still might be, one of the most abused surgical procedures in my profession. Most women, irrespective of their educational level, associate the loss of the uterus with the loss of their femininity. Even more, they believe that once this organ is lost, they'll enter menopause. They don't ask any questions about the fate of their ovaries, which are really related to fertility and menopause. When a hysterectomy is needed, I try to tell them that the uterus is only necessary to carry babies. "Just for that?" they'd say, leaving me surprised how little they know about their own genital organs. Sometimes the doctor's attitude towards the uterine problem may increase the confusion. Each doctor may recommend the treatment or procedure he's more comfortable performing. When I see doubt on a woman's face, I strongly encourage her to go for second or third opinion. She often comes back more puzzled. Some doctors recommend removing the uterus if their patient doesn't want more children; others try to convince their patient that a hysterectomy is almost always avoidable, except if malignant.

My patient was only 38 years old, had only one child, and had no bleeding or pain at that time.

"Please doctor, can you help me? I don't care if I'm done as a woman. I want my uterus removed!"

"I don't think that you need this procedure right now! You're young; there are risks. You might want another child, though."

"No way. One is enough! In fact, he's the reason I want to do it. It's a big emergency, doctor!"

I remained stone-faced, while she handed me a letter.

"Please read it."

It was a hand-written letter with the words tilted in the direction of those written by left handed people. I was busy, caught in between patients waiting outside, but I wanted to get the whole story. It was her son's letter, a young man who was deeply sorry for what he had done and was desperately asking her for help. "Mom, please help me get out of here. I feel I will die soon."

I had no inkling that she had a 19-year-old son. She started talking in a different tone: "Until last year, he was fine. He went through puberty pretty easily. I'm a single mother and started to work harder to buy a new apartment, while he fell in love with a troubled girl on drugs. She turned him upside down. By the time I figured out what was happening, his mind was gone. Then they ran away to California where he met his father: that made things worse. The girl left him; he couldn't get along with his father, and he came back home a different person. He smoked pot all day long. I had to work, so I sent him back to our country to start college. I didn't have money for college in the U.S. He seemed to be fine and came back for vacations, but then, three weeks ago, he disappeared. He left me a short letter telling me not to worry because he went to get money to start college here. "Clean money, don't worry Mom." Now he's in a Marine boot camp somewhere in California and he is desperate. He found out that from there he will go straight to Iraq or Afghanistan. He was allowed to call me yesterday from the infirmary and said that the Army is not for him. Please help, doctor!"

"I don't understand how."

"His sergeant told him that he can only be released if there is a medical emergency in his family and his help is needed, and only before he takes his oath, which is a week from now. These people aren't joking!"

A hysterectomy isn't a joke either, especially if it's not necessary. But are the over 700,000 hysterectomies performed in the U.S.A. absolutely necessary? The difference between necessary and relatively necessary is blurry when it comes to this type of procedure. Over all, my patient had a uterine fibroma which brought her to the ER, a fibroma which might grow in the coming years and give her some problems. She requested the procedure, so why shouldn't I help her? Anyhow, I didn't feel at ease because I never had to make decisions involving such circumstances. I tried something else:

"Why shouldn't we try a less invasive procedure, like cryoablation, meaning freezing the uterus, or…"

"Hysterectomy, please! The Marines are not going to release him for anything less. I need to be scheduled as soon as possible and send them proof that I had surgery and need help. I must help him, doctor! I have a bad feeling that otherwise something horrible will happen." Then she started crying.

When it comes to premonitions, Eastern European women are the worst. They could give you goose bumps because all of a sudden they get closer to the spirits and the unknown, than to logic or even God. It's difficult to handle premonitions. What if they come to fruition? In a way, she made me feel guilty in advance. I almost could see her son being hit by bullets somewhere in Afghanistan; so, I automatically picked up the phone, dialed the OR and scheduled her for a hysterectomy. She watched me with tears in her eyes. No woman had ever pushed me into the OR in such a way. Then I asked the hospital to fax me a copy with that day's schedule, I handed her a copy, and she left excited and hopeful.

Over the next few days I tried to forget the hysterectomy that I'd scheduled in such haste. I hoped that the hospital or the patient would call and let me know that something had happened and the surgery had been cancelled. It happens often enough.

The evening before surgery, just as I ended my office appointments, my assistant came in and said that one more patient had showed up. The lady with the scheduled hysterectomy came in happy. She gave me a big hug. Behind her a seven-foot-tall boy walked in, almost hitting the lintel with his head. I realized that he couldn't fit in a tank or any military vehicle, and besides, he would have been a large target. His mother was beaming. Before they left, I called the OR and told them that the hysterectomy had been cancelled.

Why?

Because her prodigal son had come back.

THE SILENT WOMAN

WHEN I WAS CALLED at the E.R., Mrs. Singh was already an established, well known patient. The resident who presented the case had an unusually quiet and indifferent voice, disproportionate to the situation's gravity. A 29-year-old woman, eight-weeks pregnant, had become paralyzed on her left side that very morning and couldn't speak anymore. I asked if she was in a coma, but she wasn't; moreover, she could communicate somehow, only that she was unable to talk. I decided to get there and examine her.

Mrs. Singh was of Indian origin, descendants from the famous tribe of Sikh warriors. The men never cut their hair and beards. Their hair, immeasurably long, is coiled around their heads and under their well-known turbans. From the age of seven, they are bound to wear a knife at all times, even if only symbolically. Since the boys have problems passing through the metal detectors in the New York schools, they are allowed to wear plastic knives, just to respect the tradition. I've never heard of any scandals or crimes involving Sikhs. Their women wear saris and seem to be less traditional than their men. In our hospital, we have three doctors with the name Singh, well respected and experienced professionals. When the operators call them on the loudspeakers, they make sure to indicate that it is doctor Singh A, B or C. They never dare to pronounce their first names because they know that would create more confusion.

Mrs. Singh was lying in bed with her eyes wide open. The first thing I noticed was the immense sadness that filled her eyes; a sadness not seen in the eyes of those who'd suffered a recent vascular accident, whose faces are usually emptied of any expression. She didn't look like a person who just had a stroke. Her left arm and leg were completely inert, and she was moving her head with difficulty. But her eyes were alive and observed all that was going on around her. I talked to her, and she understood everything, answering back with her eyes or by moving her head "yes" or "no," signs which in New York seem to be the same for everybody regardless of where they came from.

I already knew her answers, so I only asked if she wanted to keep the pregnancy. With her right hand she gestured: maybe-yes, maybe-no. I further examined her and observed, like all other doctors, that her left side was completely paralyzed, with no reflexes, non-responsive to painful stimuli. Inserting the vein catheter in her left arm didn't produce even a slight grimace from her. Before me, she'd been seen by the E.R. doctor, by the internist, neurologist and by a psychiatrist. It was pretty clear that Mrs. Sigh hadn't had a stroke, and the only certain thing we knew was that she was pregnant, so she was admitted to the gynecological department for observation. What should be "observed," wasn't clear to anybody.

The patient's sister, who had been waiting quietly, followed me out, tapped gently on my shoulder, and told me in flawless English: "You should know something, doc!"

Finally, somebody close to the patient could provide some precious information! I found out that they were immigrants from British Guyana, descendants of Indian Sikhs who had immigrated to the South American coast some two or three generations earlier. The people from British Guyana are one of the happiest folks I've ever met. I have no clue how they managed to get to that rare state of mind: happiness, on which they seem to have an unusual grasp. Most of them are Hindu, but very few practice Hinduism. They look like Indians but they are not, and have a genuine but weird sense of emancipation as they'd been taken from some Caribbean or South American island. Their joyful faces and easygoing attitudes overwhelm me like a tropical breeze that whispers in my ear that life is a beautiful game, full of giddiness and surprises. I like to work with them, but Mrs. Singh had a different look on her face. Her sister told me:

"Doc, everything started this morning, when she tried to explain something to her husband. Yesterday we went to Atlantic City, because we both like gambling. We have this vice, that's the truth. My sister had borrowed $1,000 from a relative, and she lost it all in two hours. A cousin of ours, who's a fortune teller, predicted that this particular Sunday would be her lucky day. On our way back, she said that she'd confessed to her husband that she was done with gambling. Her husband told me that this morning, over coffee, my sister tried to say something, but suddenly dropped on the floor, paralyzed and mute. Do you think it's severe?"

I knew it wasn't critical. I had almost forgotten about this malady, obviously rarer nowadays, a condition well hidden behind other names, other types of syndromes, which continue to pop up, then disappear from our medical books.

When I studied medicine in Romania, we had a course called *The History of Medicine*. It doesn't exist in American universities. I still remember the so-called lecture about the *Hysterical syndrome*, a fashionable illness, almost epidemic in the Western World at the end of the Nineteenth Century and the beginning of the Twentieth. It was during the Victorian age, when women suddenly become pale, rolled their eyes, and dropped to the floor as often and dramatically as their rank in society called for.

During those years I've learnt about the old fashion experiments done in Paris by Jean-Martin Charcot, considered the father of modern neurology, who was named "Napoleon of Neurosis." We all have in our bodies a few arteries, nerves or reflexes that bear his name. Some, less fortunate, have illnesses that carry his name. He considered hysteria a woman's issue and became famous due to his public demonstrations done in the amphitheater of the Salpetriere Hospital in Paris. Using hypnosis, he would induce a so called hysteric crisis in women. Women would be put in a trance, then the bizarre symptoms of this malady would come out one by one: convulsions, deliriums, inexplicable paralysis, sudden blindness, loss of consciousness, followed by a catatonic state.

At least Charcot came up with a new remedy, using hypnosis. Since the time of Hippocrates and Galen, the only treatment for such episodes used to be the vaginal massage and clitoris stimulation. The doctor placed a finger or two in the vagina and used to do a gentle massage on the anterior vaginal wall and clitoral area until the woman reached the so called "hysterical paroxysm." Nobody knew then about the famous and uncertain "G spot," localized, probably not by chance, on the same anterior vaginal wall. Luckily, it was "discovered" in the fifties by the German doctor E. Grafenberg who tried to present it as a new and magical island of erotic ecstasy, a spot missing on the map of women's sexuality. The controversy caused by this G spot lead to many studies and biopsies of the vagina, but its real anatomical presence remained an uncertainty, like an existent volcanic island, never truly seen.

I'm often asked by my patients to cross the border between their gynecological and their sexual problems. Many times, it's an uncomfortable crossing of a very fluid border, beyond which anything can happen. When least expected, patients may come out with surprising details of their most intimate lives and ask me peculiar questions. Maybe they just want to hear my opinion; after all, I've been their gynecologist for years. There are situations when the answer is on the tip of my tongue, but I refrain from saying it. I'm not a sexologist and I might be inclined to say that "sex is in the head," an area remote from my specialty.

Those vaginal massages could last for hours and could exhaust the patient and the doctor, or the midwife. The unmarried women were asked to get married; the married ones were told to have sex more often. A big change in this type of treatment was brought on by the discovery of electricity and the creation of the first electric vibrator in 1873, an "appliance" that had been introduced in people's home years before the vacuum cleaner or hair dryer. The famous Sears catalogue, advertising electrical devices introduced "the Vibrator" as being "very useful for home services." Its use didn't seem to have anything to do with the erotic. The vibrator is still part of the "toy box" of many modern women.

Not long ago a colleague called me to come to the Emergency Room for a private patient. The woman claimed that her vibrator had broken, and part of it remained inside her. What we found in the top of her vagina was a large 1.5 volt Duracell Ultra battery. It was easy to remove, but we called the surgeon because one of the battery electrodes produced a serious burn between the vagina and the rectum. In a few days, she developed a recto-vaginal fistula and had a long, complicated colon surgery which healed slowly and disabled her for more than a year. The woman sued the vibrator maker, but her lawyer had big headaches because the "appliance" was made in China and the lawsuit could degenerate into a strange international conflict.

Nowadays, nobody talks about hysteria anymore. At the beginning of the Twentieth Century, Freud, a student of Charcot, changed the name from hysteria to "Conversion Syndrome," trying to tie the condition to the subconscious, that part of us that we have no clue if it's ours, where it lies, what it hides, or if it works for or against us.

It's relatively easy to diagnose this condition, because the symptoms have no medical logic, appear only in certain circumstances, but can be misleading because it mimics some more serious conditions.

The next day, Mrs. Singh could slowly move her paralyzed hand, then her leg, but she still couldn't talk. Or she didn't want to. We'll never know. On the third day, I told her that we were thinking of letting her go home; then she "paralyzed" again, so she stayed in the hospital for two more days. She stood and walked only after her husband told her that he'd paid back the $1,000.

I don't know when she started talking, but in two weeks, when she came back to the office, her speech was fine. She spoke about everything but the hospital episode which she avoided as if it never happened. During the prenatal care, I saw her many times, and she would always carry a plastic cup in her hand in which she would spit often. She had strong saliva secretion, continuous and uncontrollable, which would constantly fill her mouth. She kept spiting in that cup, a habit she couldn't get rid of during the entire pregnancy.

Because Mrs. Singh had very lively, yet sad eyes, I suspected she was hiding something behind them. Some melancholy, maybe! We don't like to talk much with patients about sadness and melancholy, because then we'd have to ask for a psychiatric evaluation. In my Eastern European understanding, sadness and melancholy do not exist here, for it has been "conversely" transformed into depression.

One day, probably a melancholic day, Mrs. Singh asked me while looking to the floor, if using soap is healthy for her and her baby.

"The soap we use to wash with?" I asked.

"Yes. Only that I eat it…" she said embarrassed.

"What kind of soap?" I inquired professionally, as if the brand of soap eaten would've been of importance.

"Irish Spring, blue. It's the best, doc! I eat a bar every day…"

I was stunned, speechless. That had been my favorite soap since I'd arrived in the States. I had no clue how harmful the soap was when eaten. I hadn't learned about such things in medicine. I was quite familiar with some peculiar habits of pregnant women who eat strange things like kaolin, plaster, and now soap. Meanwhile Mrs. Singh closed the door to be sure that no one could hear us. A confessional atmosphere filled my office.

"There is something else I must tell you about this pregnancy I started eating ash…"

"What kind of ash?"

"Cigarette stuff, from ashtrays..."

"So, you're smoking while pregnant?"

"No, no! I've never smoked. Two cousins of mine, big smokers, collect it for me. Do you think it is dangerous for the baby?"

I shrugged my shoulders, resigned and helpless, completely overwhelmed by the situation. I called neither the psychiatrist nor the diet expert, and just sat there.

"Doc, when will I pass the first three months ?"

"In about a week." I said unsurely.

"Great! After three months my cravings will be gone."

She left discreetly, slowly closing the door, leaving behind a strong whiff of an ashtray mixed with Irish Spring. Following that confession, I stopped using that blue soap in my bathroom.

Mrs. Singh got over all her strange habits, except gambling. Each time she came for prenatal care, she would buy a lotto ticket from the stand across the street and bring me a cup of cappuccino. By the time she approached eight months, Mrs. Singh suddenly disappeared. I found out from another patient that she had won one of the largest jackpots, worth millions of dollars. Before she was due to deliver, she flew to Florida to give birth in a private hospital in Palm Beach, specializing in underwater deliveries. She sent a few flower bouquets, lots of ice cream, and especially for me, a large box full of Blue Irish Spring soap.

LIFE AND DEATH INSURANCE

JOE NEVER LET ME DOWN. He never stood me up financially and always gave me good advice. He's been managing my retirement money and savings since I've been a doctor in New York City, so my future has been in his hands. We call him Joe because his real name is impossible to pronounce. I only have one problem with him: he obsessed with my health, mainly with my death. Whenever we see each other, he's surprised that I'm still alive and healthy. I've asked him bluntly a few times if he has any premonition about me, and I made him roar with laughter. "Oh doctor, doctor, you are my funniest client," he always tells me. "We don't work with premonitions, we work with statistics," which sounds even more frightening. Especially when you've learnt for generations to think first about the worst case scenario and walk under a sort of Gauss curve, as if you were beneath a dome of unavoidable fatality. In this regard, Joe is worse than me because he is a professional of misfortune. Among other things, he sells all kinds of insurance, which should make you anticipate the inevitable with serenity. He constantly reminds me that every time we cross a road we may be hit by a car or a meteorite which has pierced through the stratosphere. All this on top of the ruthless ailments which can gnaw at our bodies from the inside, leaving us poor and crippled with families in despair and starving. "Oh, doctor, death is not even the worst thing that could happen to you," he would tell me when I was younger. "You can get crippled for life and be unable to do what you do best."

The idea that the sky is the limit for whoever escapes that Gauss curve is a very American metaphor, just like the more and more elusive American Dream, that we try to stuff into our filled-with-prejudices immigrant minds. Joe, who arrived in New York before me, has learnt this recipe faster. He has earned plenty of degrees in finance and investment, he knows the limits and also the boundless American sky, beyond which our dreams and our earthly remains will float, evenly and democratically. But at least he can make some money out of it.

We are both immigrants, from very different areas and tribes. I'm a Transylvanian from Romania; Joe comes from Ghana, Africa. I'm from a tribe that has suspicion and doubt engraved in its soul; he comes from a tribe whose shaman etched two knife cuts on his cheek back when he was a boy, and who initiated him in rituals of no use for him now. He must have been the son of a great chief, otherwise I cannot understand how he was able to get through and survive the whole British-American education system. He has a British accent, wears a Rolex watch, and white-starched shirts with golden cufflinks. He drives a Mercedes and always looks impeccable and in a good mood, carrying loads of papers and graphics which he will explain to you with knowledge and fairness. I see him often in my hospital when I am 'on-call,' because he has the future of many of my colleagues in his hands.

Joe works for an international company with offices on all continents, and he is passionate about his work. He is our financial advisor, our broker, so now he is a tribal chief in his own way. He comes to meetings with his younger assistants, whom he initiates in the secrets of the finest American martial arts techniques: how to make the regular Joe rich through smart investments and how to scare him to death about his life.

Back in 1996-97, Joe was carrying an old briefcase in the hospital, no Rolex, no Mercedes, no cufflinks. He kept advising us to stop investing in the stock market because we were not going to end up millionaires, as we'd thought. Nobody listened to him. We kept investing like madmen on credit, or, as they say here, "on margins," using a broker who would borrow money under our names, and would take it for a ride on the margins of a precipice which we refused to see. The stock market kept going unstoppable. The whole of America resembled a casino with demented gamblers, many of whom had quit their jobs and were involved in so-called *day-trading* from the comfort of their own homes. You could make thousands of dollars in a single day if you bought in the morning when the market opened and sold a few hours later.

Joe, who was the cousin of one of the anesthesiologists, would hang around the hospital like a herald of the Apocalypse. He grinned unconvincingly and anxiously awaited the disaster, holding his worn-out briefcase like a shield. He approached us wherever he could and asked us politely to listen to him, because he only meant well. During that time, he didn't say a word about death and illness.

When the American stock market crashed in '99, many of us went broke, lost our pensions, and were in serious debt. One doctor from Brooklyn blew his brains out. Then it was Joe who picked up our mental leftovers.

Whenever I meet up with him and he presents me with my situation, I find that my pension funds are still making the rounds in the stock market, in stocks and bonds, except that I now gamble my future cautiously. This way, if the market collapses, I fall anyway, but from a lower height. We live in a country of "gamblers," and Joe now tells me that the greatest risk of my life can come from illnesses, car accidents, and meteorites.

"So, you told me you go skiing! Well, let me tell you what happened to a surgeon from Colorado on his last descent of his unfortunate holiday..."

"Oh, Joe, don't start again with your examples!"

Otherwise, my colleagues and I are pleased with him. He guides us with a sure hand, but slowly, and keeps us safely invested by scaring us to death. He presents reports, facts and graphics, and eventually gets to the nothingness that will, one day, absorb us without mercy. Every meeting with Joe ends with being scolded for not being sufficiently protected against the dangers that I face with every step. If I roll my eyes or seem absent-minded, he begins again to recount all the wounded and the dead he knew personally, and the conversation becomes quite unbearable.

When I was younger, I witnessed illnesses and severe accidents which could have made me psychologically incapable of working in a hospital. Joe didn't let me off the hook until I signed a disability policy which insured all my vital organs, my heart, my brain, and especially my very important hands, with all their ten fingers. Without them I could not perform surgery anymore. I tried to save money by wriggling out of at least one or two fingers, by telling him I was not a pianist, what the heck, but it didn't work. Dismemberment insurance stipulates how much I would receive if I lost one, two, or three fingers, one hand or both, plus my legs, one at a time. Legs are cheaper. For every possibility, Joe had plenty of real-life examples, which made your hair stand up.

Oh God, I can't refrain from remembering what a carefree life we lived in Romania in the old days. We smoked without remorse; we carelessly ate bacon and fried lard with no fear of cholesterol or cancer. We drove on decrepit roads with unbuckled safety belts, and no meteorites ever fell from the sky. The future was small and grim, we knew that, but we couldn't care less, and we looked with serenity at the sky, not thinking that *the sky is the limit*. I know that anxiety, as well as life and death insurance, now exist in Romania as well. In 1993, when I returned to Romania for the first time, I witnessed capitalism, instituting itself rapidly, wildly and chaotically. One evening, a salesman who seemed to have come out of the America of the '50s or '60s, visited the relatives I was staying with. He came to their home to sell them a fantastic vacuum cleaner that picked up everything, absolutely everything. He began his pitch by showing my relatives a few grotesque images made under a microscope that magnified all the germs, protozoans and roaches that lived in their home and in their lungs. And the salesman convinced them: they were ready to pay thousands of dollars for a mediocre vacuum cleaner.

I continued to pay hundreds of dollars a month for years and years for my dismemberment insurance, until I got close to 60 and noticed that I still had all my fingers. Then Joe announced that after age 65, insurance would not pay me anything in case I suffered all the calamities that didn't come to pass. Suddenly our discussions switched to my inevitable death. I did have life insurance, but he convinced me to increase it, because in case something… there wouldn't be much left when I am gone. He spoke about my family, how they shouldn't have to suffer after my passing, but on the contrary…. I wonder what he meant by "on the contrary." I asked him again if he had any premonitions, because I trusted his African instinct. He answered with a slightly eerie laugh, and resorted again to statistics and overwhelming real-life examples.

I am not sure why, but every time I now pass by the hospital morgue, I think about Joe. I pay a lot of money every year. I admit that this money is not entirely lost as it is with dismemberment insurance, because Joe makes smart investments with it and, after all, I can take out some of it, if I get out alive from this whole ordeal that no one knows how long will last. I have a special, very good insurance policy that Joe offers only to his oldest, most devoted clients, who have withstood him for many years. Long live Joe!

Lately he's been telling me "look, the life expectancy for males has increased, so you are healthy and well, doctor." He then adds that the greatest risk for us (he always uses the plural) is for us to live too long, and end up so old and impaired as to not be able to take care of ourselves. It's true that my father, God bless him, has reached and surpassed the age of 90! My father still travels, reads, writes poems for a new book, he has plans for the future! If I get to his age, or even further, who will take care of me? I try to suggest to Joe that I might do what my father did: hire a young, strong woman who will cook, wash, take good care of me with no damn term life insurance. With that, I offended him a bit. He seemed upset for a moment, but then gave me his shamanic smile and whispered: "Don't fool yourself, doctor! In twenty years from now the price for such a woman will increase tremendously. You come from the

European Community, don't you?" You can't win with Joe. You can only buy more insurance.

Now Joe tries to convince me to set up a life policy for my wife as well, and, why not, even for our children. They are adults, all grown up, it can happen to them too, and then I will at least get something after I took care of them. The wife smokes? Yes, my wife smokes and she doesn't want to quit. That's good and bad at the same time, Joe whispers almost imperceptibly. The life insurance is a little more expensive, but it is worth it. Smoking is so dangerous!

I remembered a case which had been all over the media, about a murderer who insured his entire family, including the dog, locked all of them up inside the house, used carbon dioxide to make them fall asleep, and then set them on fire. Ouch!

"You travel a lot doctor," Joe continued undaunted. "You fly a lot, and you never know. You might both be gone at once, and then the children could live well, at peace. Maybe you have family inheritances... We have a policy which stipulates that in case of a fatal accident, we can establish which of you died first, you or your wife, depending on what is more convenient for the two of you. This ensures that there will be no disputes in the family about who inherits from whom and what. We are very flexible, doctor!" Then he adds, gently and professionally: "I get the feeling that your mind is somewhere else right now. We will discuss more next time." Joe noticed that he'd lost me, and during such a moment, he wordlessly drew charts for me on paper until my eyes got tired and teary.

The years are going by, I am approaching retirement and life goes on, indifferent, careless and busy. I now meet with Joe less often because my money is nodding out in the same low-risk stocks and almost inexistent profit, and he has nothing left to sell me. I always took from him what I thought made sense. I listened to him every time, and in the end he never tried to push too aggressively.

"The stock market is not going well, doctor, and neither is the world in general," he told me during our most recent meeting, displaying the same shamanic smile.

"Do you have some bad premonitions, Joe?"

So—so, his body language said.

He stopped offering me any kind of insurance, and advised me to be careful with my money. We know what kind of world we live in. Now we just drink coffee together and talk about life, both of us careless and fearless. He has a sense of humor and is curious. He always asks me what I am writing. And that's how I got the idea!

"Joe, what would you say if the two of us created a new insurance? Not a life insurance, but one for the afterlife, for after death? Karma is included as a clause. We'll call it *Afterlife Insurance*! What do you think?"

Joe roared with laughter. "Oh, doctor, doctor, you truly are my funniest client." Then he paused, wiped away his tears, and told me calmly and professionally: "You know, it's not such a silly idea after all. I'm sure we'll find some buyers."

BIG TROUBLE

WOMEN WHO HAVE DIMPLES in their cheeks age gracefully. Even when they get older, age doesn't give them away because those happy dimples in their cheeks seem to swallow up the tough years piled up on their backs.

Felicia was only 33 and still had an air of joyful-healthy youthfulness. Besides her dimples, she continuously smiled with her eyes, a woman born with a good nature who spread a contagious good aura all around her. When she came in for prenatal care, in just a few seconds, she would change the whole mood in my office. She was a sweet and relaxed talker, with a casual natural humor as if she'd known everybody for a while. She always came alone to the office, so I couldn't associate the image of the child I was observing on the ultrasound screen with that of the man who would be his father. I asked her once where her husband was, and she said that he worked so much that even she didn't get to see him often.

I saw him only at the time of birth; a thin young man, not too tall, with lots of tattoos on his body, judging by the ones that were revealed by his rolled-up sleeves or were snaking up his neck. He'd come from an Eastern European country when he was four years old and seemed to have become Americanized from head to toe. Like most people who immigrated when they were very young, he couldn't remember anything of the place where he'd been born. All he and others like him knew came from the boring stories their parents, who continued to speak a foreign language at home, told them. They also could only use a few, dry words of their birth language, connecting them like old laundry hanging on a rope between mother and father.

In the last two months of pregnancy, Felicia kept talking to her baby girl who surely must have heard and understood what she was saying. Although she'd been living in America for quite some time, she spoke to her baby in her native language.

"I want her to speak in my mother-tongue too, although I know that's a tall order," she said.

One night, Felicia called me at home because her water broke. That was nothing unusual for me, but not when she said that she could hear her baby girl crying inside her. There was a long pause in our conversation, until I suddenly woke up because the news that an unborn baby was crying in the belly of one of my patients put me in a strange state of unease.

Felicia wasn't the type of person to talk nonsense. This was a situation that I'd never encountered. Although anecdotally possible, it had not been described in any obstetrical book. I couldn't tell her that she was talking nonsense, because an unborn baby *can* cry inside the mother's belly if the water is broken and air gets inside the uterus. A baby cannot cry unless he breathes air in his lungs. I heard about such unusual cases, but never in my thirty years of practice had I heard a child cry before being born. I quickly ran to the hospital.

I am not certain that Felicia's baby girl had truly cried before birth, because once in the hospital nothing abnormal happened. Twice, they called me to the Delivery Room to hear the cries of the unborn baby, but I couldn't hear anything. Only the Resident that was 'on-call' that night said that she heard something. She was a short woman, very thin, originally from south India, where women during Hindu holidays would temporarily tattoo their hands and fingers with nice filigree forms.

But Felicia certainly did hear something, because in the end that was her child, still inside her body. Her husband was silent, very silent, almost indifferent to our dilemma of the baby crying. When the baby's heartbeat lowered, I examined her and had the impression that I could hear a strange cry coming from her belly, as if it came from a deep cave.

The baby's heart recovered quickly, and I knew she was ready to come into this world. When Felicia started to push, her husband's face turned pale. She let go of his hand and asked him to wait outside until all was over.

"He's too sensitive," said Felicia. "I don't want him to pass out and give you a problem!"

Felicia behaved well while giving birth, as she probably did in all difficult situations she went through. The labor pains cast some shadows across her face, but after she got an epidural, those cheek-dimples came back and her face lit up again. I knew that she'd been waiting a long time for the moment to give birth. As soon as the baby was out, the girl started to cry at the top of her lungs, and Felicia was crying with happiness. I wanted to call her husband in to cut the umbilical cord, but she stopped me.

"Let him wait outside, please. I don't want him to see me like this!" She still had the placenta inside and was bleeding slightly which called for sutures because I had to make a little incision on her perineum to avoid a larger laceration.

"Doctor, I don't think men should witness all this," Felicia continued calmly. "If I were a man, I'd be waiting outside until everything is over. This mess might curb his desire to go to bed with me. My grandmother used to say that we're born between urine and feces, and so it is."

I nodded in agreement. I saw situations when men were pushed by family and wives to stay and witness the whole birthing process, even though they would have preferred to wait outside. Felicia seemed to be a very accommodating woman, trying to protect her husband and her own sexuality.

Some women who come for a simple gynecological exam bring in their husbands because the men think they can assist at the vaginal exam, which seems pretty odd to me. Some women want to show that they have nothing to hide, or the husband is a jealous person, who doesn't like the doctor intimately examining his wife.

Women who are dominated by authoritarian husbands want their men to be part of all the suffering that comes with the birthing process. Giving birth is a triumphant moment, a rare chance to show the tyrant what it really means to be a woman, and the pains they have to endure. Some women scream, pull or pinch the man's arm, even bully him a bit, without fear of reprisal. What man would dare be a jerk or behave badly with his wife there who is giving birth to his progeny? Felicia's husband didn't belong to this category. After everything ended in the Delivery Room, I looked at them carefully. He seemed completely overwhelmed by the whole situation. When I left, the baby girl was quietly nursing at her mother's breast, and Felicia was smiling with a happy face while he was taking pictures.

Three months later, she came to my office because she wanted to have an intrauterine device implanted for contraception. She didn't want anything hormonal because she was trying to lose weight. During her pregnancy she'd gained some extra pounds, but the pounds didn't show because she was tall and muscular. In her youth she'd been a good swimmer.

"I look like a whale! Don't I?" She asked smiling

It wasn't so, but I did encourage her to use a copper intrauterine device, which wouldn't make her gain weight. I examined her and did cervical cultures and everything seemed to be just fine. She brought me a photo of her baby girl which I placed in the gallery of "my" babies that stretches along the wall in the waiting room of my office.

A few days later, I got the results, and I had to call her back because one of the tests was abnormal. I saw her the same week, and for the first time I noticed that her dimples and smile on her face had disappeared. I explained what I'd found out and told her that Chlamydia was a venereal disease and her husband needed treatment also.

"Is it the one with crosses in the blood?" she asked sternly.

I told her it wasn't, suddenly remembering the syphilis of bygone days and the Wasserman test, when the "crosses in the blood" counted, indicating how positive the test was.

"Is this a kind of American gonorrhea?" she tried once more.

"Something like that. Only it's a different kind of bacteria that's treated with antibiotics."

"I didn't have it when I was pregnant."

That was truly the case. I had tested her a few months earlier, and the test came out negative. I gave her a prescription for her and her husband. Then she quietly took the baby in her arms, and before she left, asked me to give her a copy of the results.

She came back in two weeks to get tested again. She was very quiet, troubled and ashamed about the whole affair. The results came in fine, and when I told her this, a smile came back to her face. The sadness went away like a summer's rain.

"Did he take the medication?" I asked.

"How else! I told him that if he didn't, I'd punch him again."

"You hit him?"

"Hard enough. As soon as I got home, I asked my mother-in-law to hold the baby and handed him the Chlamydia results. I don't know how much he managed to see because I put him down with one single blow. When he recovered, I just told him 'Dirty scum. I've never been so embarrassed in my whole life. Maybe that's why my baby girl was crying inside me…'"

"Wow! He didn't hit you back?"

"He didn't have a chance with me, Doc! I have a heavy hand, trust me. I beat him up badly. I called 'Chlamydia' right away, because I know who she is, and told her that I'll break her legs if I ever see her close to my man. Now it's a closed case. It's not cancer, so it isn't worth holding much anger and bitterness in our hearts!"

THE STRIPED ELEPHANT

MY LAWYER SPOKE SLOWLY and emphatically, avoiding my eyes as if he didn't want me to see what lay behind his words. It's difficult to look at a victim straight in the eyes while trying to tell him that he doesn't have much of a chance. He was staring at his well shined shoes while playing with a Mont Blanc pen, which I'm sure he had received as a gift from some company promoting products made for attorneys, just like doctors are often given such gifts by pharmaceutical companies.

I was taking notes with a pen which advertised a new vaginal lubricant. To me, the attorney represented the law itself—an institution that I respected, an ancient invention, still slippery like wet soap in the bathroom.

"My advice is to settle! They're not asking for much. When you were summoned, they wanted two million dollars, now they'd accept $250,000. Better do it now, before we get deeper into the trial," he said, while sketching a few lines onto his yellow pad, lines which started to look like the profile of the bartender who was standing in front of us. My lawyer seemed to have a real gift for drawing.

It was lunch time, and we were seated in a restaurant right across from the Queens Court in New York. My appetite had disappeared completely. The millions that I was supposed to pay in damages got stuck in my throat like large bones, even if they now transformed into hundreds of thousands dollars. It was a sunny May day, and we'd just gotten through the first court appearance.

The plaintiff's furious lawyer introduced me to the nine jurors and the judge as a criminal, pointing at me in utter indignation, foaming at the mouth. His diatribe was only the hysteric overture of the tragi-comic masquerade that was to come in the next three weeks. That first day of trial outraged me so much and gave me such a bad taste that I had the impulse to give up and settle. No matter how much I had to pay, as long as I didn't have to go back to that court room.

The plaintiff's attorney, a tall man almost six-foot-eight, imposing and cold, began accusing the hospital first, which he described as a madhouse, a dangerous place where a doctor, a Resident, or a midwife would irresponsibly put your life and your child in danger.

The mother of the harmed child, a woman of about thirty-five, was quietly flipping through a fashion magazine. The boy who I supposedly hurt at birth, a pretty and joyful kid, was sitting in a chair beside his mom, unhappily swinging his legs. He seemed to be a cheery healthy kid, whom I delivered under dramatic circumstances almost five years earlier. Clearly brought to court against his wishes, the child started moving around, trying to play. Obviously, he would have rather played at home or watched TV. I couldn't have recognized him and didn't even remember his mother because a pregnant woman who's giving birth is an altogether different person than the one you see every day. She wasn't my private patient, and I saw her for the first time during an 'on-call', a few hours before she delivered.

"If you settle today, it's all over. That's why you have insurance. What do you think, doctor?"

I shook my head in disagreement. He continued to sketch the bartender's portrait which was almost finished. It looked pretty well done, but he drew the man's Adam's apple too large, as if it was his most prominent feature.

"Why should I pay? Did you see the boy? He looks fine and healthy."

"I saw him! Still, we have no clue what surprises they might bring in what their experts will say!"

The boy, who had been sitting quietly in his chair for almost an hour, began to lose patience. At some point he turned his head towards me as if he was curious to see what kind of doctor had brought him into the world. I smiled at him and discreetly gestured with my hand. He smiled back. The child couldn't grasp what was really happening and got off his chair to start playing in the court room. He would turn his head and look at me as neglected kids do in need of reassurance. I carefully observed the way he moved, particularly his hands, which he used normally and efficiently. This was the victim of my so called medical negligence, for which I was being asked to pay lots of money in damages.

If I don't write about my lawsuits and my fear of practicing in the U.S., it would be as if I were ignoring the striped elephant that is roaming daily through our hospitals and offices, a hungry and strange house-trained animal, who's getting wilder and more untamable. We don't know how the hell he got into our house and we can't get rid of him anymore. An elephant with whom we must get used to, learn how to outsmart and professionally avoid.

In the beginning I believed that the fear of being sued was just one of those American myths that existed only in theory—a hypothetical and transparent elephant that would not trample you as long as you did the right thing. I was coming from a country where everything was permitted and forbidden at the same time. We played a game with no precise rules. In Romania, it was almost inconceivable to be sued as a doctor, even if you were at fault, because mistakes could happen and were accepted. A doctor was considered a little God back then. In the U.S., a doctor cannot work a single day unless insured for malpractice. My malpractice insurance doubled in about 15 years. The increase in my insurance wasn't because of lawsuits. The cost of malpractice insurance in New York is one of the highest in the U.S. One of the reasons is that we have the largest concentration of lawyers and law firms per capita, which has created a Pavlovian reflex to sue. Lawyers are constantly on the watch, and even if you have no intention of suing, if a case comes up, somebody could tap you on the shoulder, whisper in your ear, convince you that award settlements for troubles and unfortunate events are handsomely paid in the U.S. Money, money! The magic word of the world we live in.

Two years earlier, when my car was hit from behind, even before the ambulance showed up, somebody handed me the business card of a lawyer specializing in auto accidents. Those who specialize in malpractice are far more aggressive. Very expensive ads run on all the major TV channels, day and night. They always find a new way to squeeze money from doctors, hospitals, drug companies, or companies that manufacture instruments and medical products.

Naval yards, construction sites, and every place where asbestos had been used for construction are still haunted by lawsuits many years after asbestos became illegal. The famous "mesothelioma" ad has been continuously running day and night on all

TV channels for many years: "Do you have mesothelioma, or know anybody who has it? Call our firm right away! You may be entitled to a large financial compensation." As the cases of mesothelioma become rarer and are probably caused by other factors, these ads become more excessive and pathetic.

Mesothelioma is a rare pulmonary or digestive cancer, and the asbestos, used in the past for insulation, was considered one of the causes. The same asbestos that insulated the stoves used for heating in my youth, next to which I slept for years. It's known that the U.S. government had placed billions of dollars in an escrow fund, just to settle these cases of mesothelioma. The lawyers are going nuts and constantly looking for new cases because there are not many left. Time goes by, and the money sits there for nothing. "Please come out of the closet and be diagnosed with mesothelioma!", the TV ads are almost begging! "We'll prove that some asbestos existed in your life, somewhere, sometime, somehow. Do not suffer in silence! We're here for you!" These are desperate advertisements. Payments in the order of tens of millions of dollars are guaranteed for each case.

Every month I see new ads on TV, blaming contraceptives, or other FDA approved good drugs, that are now accused of killing people. No doctor dares to prescribe that medication anymore, even when patients ask for it. All it takes is for the public to hear about a few bizarre side effects and the lawsuits begin. They do not seek justice. It's only about money, calculated attack, calculated defense. It's true that in the process something good might come out of it, like the case against cigarette smoking.

In the last two years a new ad was launched on TV. Two large law firms were specializing in possible complications linked to new synthetic slings and meshes used in surgery treating genital prolapse and urinary incontinence. I have done many such surgeries with good results, but after seeing the ads for the law firms, I've stopped doing them, and lots of gynecologists in the U.S. have dropped these new procedures. This good sling-mesh-procedure, invented in Sweden, reached the U.S.A. in the late '90s, only after it was tested successfully for almost ten years on millions of women, in Europe, Asia, and South America. Good-bye, slings and meshes!

On the other hand, CNN uncovered that in 2013, in the U.S.A., there were over thirty cases weekly when instruments and other materials were simply forgotten in the bodies of patients who had been operated on, thirty cases when an operation was performed on the wrong side of the patient's body, and thirty others that were performed incorrectly. All this is happening today, even with all the strict protocols in the Operating Rooms. To err is human, but in America, no mistake is accepted. The reporter advised pragmatically and candidly that patients who have a fever after surgery should ask their surgeon: "Listen doctor, did you forget something inside me?" When you are a Resident, you are less aware of these dangers because you work under a hospital's license, covered by a specialist who's responsible for everything. Not long ago a new patient who came to the Delivery Room, looked coldly at my ID badge and asked: "What kind of name is that?"

"Romanian," I responded smiling. "Why do you ask?"

"To remember, if I have to take you to court!"

She wasn't kidding.

In my last year of Residency, I was called for the first time to give a deposition for a large law firm in Manhattan. The deposition lasted from ten in the morning to five in the afternoon. I left the place with an awful headache and a firm conviction that the striped elephant truly exists.

That law suit was the result of a tragic case. A nineteen-year-old girl had died in childbirth. Nobody did anything wrong, but the situation was out of the ordinary. She was a young African American woman who suffered from Sickle Cell disease, a genetic condition found only in those descending from Africa. The girl had a severe form that was further aggravated by pregnancy. On top of this, she'd stopped going for prenatal care after her first trimester of pregnancy when she was told about all the risks. The crisis of Sickle Cell disease is due to the massive destruction of the defective red blood cells. The failing of vital organs can occur rapidly, and the patient might die.

That young woman had simply disappeared from medical care until she was very close to term. She was brought in by the ambulance in severe crisis, looking like moribund. The baby was still fine, but the mother's heart was giving in rapidly. The Attending 'on-call' was a specialist in high risk pregnancies, and the patient was carefully treated by a full team of anesthesiologists and intensive care specialists. The idea was to stabilize her, then do a caesarian in order to get the baby out fast and safely. We had to take care of two lives within the same body. She had been resuscitated but her heart and kidneys had given up and she developed a massive pulmonary edema. It was past six o'clock in the evening when I heard the loudspeakers blasting *Code 99* in the Delivery Room and ran in that direction. I'd already signed out and was dressed in street clothes, ready to head home. *Code 99* means that a patient's heart has stopped. It was the first case of severe Sickle Cell disease that I have ever seen, but I was experienced in doing urgent and fast caesarian sections. The patient's heart stayed still after four or five attempts at C.P.R. The sharp-monotonous beep of the monitor lashed our ear drums, a siren of death. My Attending, with whom I had worked closely for three years, was doing C.P.R. and shouted at me over the others' heads: "Get the baby out. Fast!"

When the mother is dying, an urgent caesarian must be done as quickly as possible, to save the child who might still be alive. The scalpel was already in my hand. I'd barely removed my wristwatch and put gloves on, while somebody else rolled up my shirt sleeves. I never got to an unborn so fast. A very dark liquid was slowly oozing from the wound because her heart had stopped pumping. I cut the uterus with care, trying not to hurt the baby, whom I extracted in a few seconds and whose cry tempered the sorrowful sound of the monitors.

"Did you apply iodine on the mother's belly before the incision? Speak up doctor, did you use iodine?" This was one of the questions the plaintiff's attorney asked loudly. I remembered that somebody did apply iodine on the patient's belly, because when I got home, it had stained my shirt and pants.

That day, as I was suturing back the girl's uterus, something strange happened. Suddenly, blood started to flow, then gush, changing its color from black to red. I never enjoyed seeing pouring blood, but that time, blood meant life was coming back to a dead body! A shot of adrenaline was administered in the heart, and after I did cardiac massage through her diaphragm, the woman's heart began suddenly to pump again. The girl came back to life and lived fully for three more days. Unfortunately, she developed a severe postpartum cardiomyopathy and all her vital organs collapsed. The cardiologist said that even an urgent heart transplant couldn't have saved her. She'd been conscious all the time and kept asking: "What happened? Where's my baby?"

When I saw her after surgery, I introduced myself and told her that I was the one who delivered her baby.

"I know; I saw when you did it!"

I stood perplexed for a moment, certain that she could not have seen me, because she had been put to sleep, intubated, and in a state of clinical death.

"How could you have seen me? From where?" I asked bluntly.

"I saw you and heard you! From where I was! You put your wrist watch in your chest pocket. It almost fell inside me when you leaned forward... I could hear it ticking!"

At that moment, I was deeply touched by her words, but not for long. You cannot think too much about such things, certainly not in a Delivery Room where life and death hovers above us like nowhere else. During my deposition I remembered that surreal moment, surrounded by a few very real lawyers. I would have liked to have seen how they'd react to such a story, to see if their faces furrowed, marked by the blades of law and righteousness, but I didn't say anything.

The long and inquisitorial deposition convinced me, without falling into any paranoia, that behind us, there was a whole system that was watching. After hours of madly repetitive questioning, I understood that they were trying to find, or create a little crack in my deposition, only to get to where they wanted to go. Meaning money! All the procedures performed that day in the hospital had been done correctly, though desperately. No one had mentioned that the baby had been saved. Later on, I found out that one of the other defendants had made some small mistakes which he admitted in his deposition, so that the hospital and the Attending responsible for the case had decided to settle even before the case was brought to court. I don't know how much of that money went toward the child's education. For sure over a third of the settlement went into the attorneys' pockets.

It was then that I remembered the critical situations I'd encountered in Romania where no lawsuits were ever imposed on doctors. That wasn't right either! It was a society that did not protect the patient's interests, and doctors were only held responsible when caught making mistakes of excessive gravity. Even then there were only minor repercussions.

"No, I don't want to settle! I had done nothing wrong, and the baby was perfectly fine," I told my attorney who had finished the bartender's portrait and started to show some interest in my facial features. He looked at me for a while and said:

"OK, doctor! You have a fifty-fifty chance, and it's your right to defend yourself. But, we must prepare this seriously!"

He said it in such a solemn tone, as if we had to prepare ourselves for an expedition into a jungle full of danger and surprises. He knew what he was talking about!

In the next few weeks we got to know each other quite well, and my respect for his profession grew. Other depositions followed in the court, and we had to prepare for them for hours and hours. We had a few meetings in the backyard of my house, right under the kitchen's window, where my wife, who kept making tea, could hear us. We had countless cups of tea, gallons of mineral water, and would take turns running to the toilet while my blood pressure was sky high. Each time I went into the house, I'd find my wife terrified, holding her face in her hands:

"For God's sake! You shouldn't allow him to talk to you like that!" she would say.

I wasn't aware that he was doing anything wrong. My lawyer, with all his rough-tough talking, had been smartly taking on the plaintiff's attorney's role. He tried to prepare me for the worst, helping me to develop some anticipative immunity, some resilience to the under-the-belt punches he knew I was going to get. He was right. Once in the court room, it was like being in a boxing ring where all I could do was avoid the punches by smart foot play and a little reflex thinking. I would have made lots of mistakes without the mock trial we had in my backyard.

Overnight, the plaintiff's attorney had turned into a sort of specialist in vacuum assisted deliveries and shoulder dystocia. That was the accusation I was facing: he claimed that by using the vacuum extraction at the birth, I'd caused the blocking of the shoulder and damaged one hand. The Vacuum Extractor is a pretty atraumatic instrument which had replaced the forceps at delivery, a quite dangerous instrument which I'd used often in the past. I'd used the vacuum to extract the baby's head because it had gotten stuck in the mother's pelvis; the baby's heart was beating low, and the mother was exhausted and couldn't push any more. The vacuum had been created for just such situations. The head came out easily, but the shoulder had gotten blocked.

Shoulder dystocia is always an unexpected complication, and once it occurs, it can become more aggravated by the minute. If not treated fast and appropriately, the baby and the mother could suffer serious complications. Trying all kinds of maneuvers one by one, I managed to get the baby out in time, and his Apgar score was excellent, except that one of his hands was moving poorly, a minor form of paresis, common in such cases, which resolved completely in the next four weeks.

The plaintiff's attorney claimed money compensation for the newborn and his mother's suffering, without mentioning that I might have saved the baby from something potentially far more dangerous.

My first deposition was fine, and my lawyer was happy that I stepped in on the right foot, as if I were tiptoeing on land mines. I believe he didn't expect that an Eastern European like me, with an accent and difficulties in understanding the legal terms and the intricacies of the American justice system, would play his role so well. My deposition lasted for two full days as it was a complicated crime. To each of the accusatory questions, I was supposed to answer 'yes' or 'no'. I felt as if each 'yes' and 'no' had taken on the steps of a monosyllabic dwarf which little by little would bring me closer to a trap. My victory came when the judge allowed me to explain my answers in addition to the 'yes' or 'no', which infuriated the plaintiff's attorney.

An infuriated accuser looks like a mace-brandishing troll, and the little boy whom we were fighting for, felt his anger, got scared, and wasn't brought in for the second day. He had lost his patience, as any child with a healthy mind would have done. He'd begun to play throughout the court room and even tried to get up on the judge's table. The judge, a man of almost retirement age, paid attention to all the details and a few times stressed that the accuser was going too far.

Then came the plaintiff's expert, a doctor who claimed to be an ex-Harvard professor. His role was a difficult one because he was a colleague of mine who'd been paid to damage my professional reputation. He played the saddest part in this whole spectacle. I glanced over his biography and understood it all. He used to be some kind of professor, but stopped practicing years before and now was selling his expertise. During lunch break, my lawyer told me bluntly:

"They're ready to settle for one hundred and fifty thousand dollars. You never know how things could turn…"

"I'm not budging!"

"OK, then. Let's move forward!"

Two more mock sessions followed in my backyard. My wife was getting used to my lawyer's aggressive style and would bring him cups of calming tea.

"Why such a circus?" I dared ask him at some point. "The mother is well; the boy is fine… How long will it last?"

"I don't know! I warn you, they will become more vicious. The firm has already spent lots of money," he said.

My malpractice insurance was paying him by the hour, so as the expenses were mounting, so was to the pressure to settle.

During a break before the final court appearance, I told him the story of Princess Charlotte of Wells in England and Sir Richard Croft, the royal obstetrician, who in 1817 took care of the princess during her first pregnancy and assisted her at birth. I looked at my attorney's face, which was expressionless and described how after Dr. Croft had made the princess go hungry during the last months of pregnancy and bled her, which was the custom of the times for pretty much everything, he assisted her during delivery. The princess was in labor for over fifty hours in her own bedroom. After two days of incredible pain, she gave birth to a stillborn baby boy weighing over 9 pounds, who would have been the inheritor of England's throne. Sir Croft had avoided the use of forceps during that difficult birth, an instrument that had fallen in disgrace. The vacuum had not yet been discovered, and a caesarian was not feasible. The princess, who would have become the Queen of

England, died five hours later, most likely because of internal bleeding. King George the Fourth ordered the princess' autopsy and declared Sir Croft free of all charges.

The case remained known in history as "the triple obstetrical tragedy" because Croft could not live with such a failure and put a bullet through his head.

"Tough," mumbled my lawyer blankly. Then I tested his endurance, telling the story of a New Jersey pathologist whom I had known. He hung himself the morning he had to go to court for a misdiagnosed case of breast cancer.

"That's even tougher," said the attorney dryly.

"In the U.S. there are 300-400 suicides among doctors annually, most of them being psychiatrists, ophthalmologists and obstetricians," I said. These facts were well known to my attorney as well, but he didn't seem eager to talk about them.

"Why so many ophthalmologists?" I asked him.

"Doc, I have no clue! I specialize in cases involving obstetrics and gynecology. Let's get back to our case, please!"

My trial went on for two more weeks. I had to call the hospital to get some days off, reduced my clinic hours, and cancelled a few surgeries. The company which insured me, as well as my hospital that paid for it, kept pressuring me to settle. Had I lost the case, the insurance company would have paid lots more, same as my hospital, which was also being sued. Then I found out that my hospital had settled separately. Now the lawyers could focus solely on me. I decided to go all the way.

Six years earlier I had made the mistake of settling before trial. It was the first lawsuit against me, and I'd been intimidated too easily. Technically, that case was far more than I could handle. One morning, when I was taking over the 'on-call' shift, I stupidly caught "an unpinned hand grenade that blew in your face, doc."

Those were the exact words of my attorney back then. While we were signing out the patients, a woman gave birth to her first twin who was fine and whose umbilical cord was being tied.

"How is the second baby?" I asked.

My colleague, who had allowed the woman to give birth naturally, had examined her and told me that the second baby was in transverse lie, meaning horizontal in the uterus, a fetal position incompatible with a vaginal birth. In the U.S., the manual extraction of the second twin through internal version was considered too risky, as it was delivery in breech, when the baby comes out butt first. In Romania doctors delivered, naturally, breech presentations, but the extraction of the second twin through caesarian was inconceivable. Once the first twin was born naturally, the second could be extracted manually regardless of its position. I had done that many times, but in the U.S. this wasn't recommended. My colleague, tired after that night, asked me if I would do the cesarean section. I mumbled a bit, but I took the woman to the Operating Room. I scrubbed fast but no anesthesiologist was around. He showed up ten minutes later, a very precious ten minutes.

The baby came out with a low Apgar score, but recovered well. When I removed the placenta, I saw that it was almost decollated after the birth of the first twin, nearly choking the second baby. I was sued a year later, when the second twin started having neurological problems. After three years, I had the first pretrial deposition when I was told that the boy had been "damaged." It was my shortest deposition, less than half an hour, and I left convinced that I was off the hook. It wasn't me who'd made the decision to let the first twin come out naturally, and when I took over, the situation was already set. But the "grenade" exploded in my hand.

One year later, I was informed that my colleague had retired and had gone back to Philippines. Five years after that delivery, my attorney called me and advised me to settle. While he was talking to me, he wasn't looking in my eyes and was also drawing something on a yellow pad—sketching perfect circles that were intersecting strangely and looked very abstract. He seemed like an aspiring postmodern artist.

"You shouldn't have taken the case," he said dryly. "I don't want to remind you of the hand grenade with the pin removed."

We didn't see the damaged child, but the plaintiff's expertise report showed that he displayed "neurological damage."

"If he does have serious problems and they bring him in a wheelchair, you might come out much worse than if you settle now!"

I wanted to take the case to trial but my attorney said the same thing: "You have a 50/50 chance, which is not good enough!"

I felt cornered, and in the end I settled. My insurance premium didn't increase. It was all taken care of between the lawyers who were negotiating among themselves, while most likely drawing lines on their yellow pads. If my insurance rose, or I settled many times, I could have been dropped by the hospital and the insurance company. I knew that "next time" I'd have to fight.

I saw the twins three years later when their mother came back to the hospital to have another baby. They both seemed fine.

The case with the vacuum and shoulder dystocia had reached its final phase. Our expert testified better than their expert, because he was not a professor, but a real obstetrician still delivering babies. The plaintiff's attorney became more furious, more caustic and stopped looking as tall. I was present during the entire trial because I wanted to see and absorb everything. The amount of human energy, money, ambition and wasted time was incredible. The idea of justice itself had disappeared completely in an obscure fog, and the jury understood that the case was all about money.

A case like this wouldn't have been accepted by a court of law anywhere else in the world. Many American states would have rejected it as being "frivolous." Nine American citizens had been doing their jury duty and were brought in the court room daily to judge my "crime." There were six women and three men, most of them Caribbean immigrants, as was the woman I delivered. The morning of the sentence, the plaintiff's attorney asked the judge to allow him to interrogate me one more time. That was after my lawyer did his job and conveyed to me that they were willing to settle for just thirty-five thousand dollars.

Five other lawyers from the same large Manhattan firm showed up that day, somber and determined like strange commandos, dressed in black suits and ties, holding their familiar yellow pads in their hands. That small trial became for them an issue of reputation and pride. I was called to the stand. The tall lawyer accused me of the same old things, spewing saliva on the jurors whom he wanted to somehow hypnotize.

In response to all the questions, my attorney screamed "objection," a nice word that still rings in my ears. In the end, the plaintiff's attorney got really mad and suddenly moved his hand to his breast pocket. I thought he'd pull out a pistol and order me to "give up, damn it!" To everybody's surprise, he pulled out a vacuum extractor, like the one I used in the hospital. He presented it to the jurors as an instrument of torture from the days of the Inquisition; then he applied it to his hand with the vacuum cup tightly squeezed, and started to remove the air, creating the vacuum that makes the extraction of the fetus' head possible. He was trying to convince the jury that the mark left on his hand was nothing compared to the possible damages to a newborn, damages which could show up years later, during school, college, or the army. All of a sudden, the vacuum became like a strange gun with delayed effects. The demonstration became pathetic, because he didn't know how to apply the vacuum to his hairy hand.

When I volunteered my own head, the judge, who'd reached a point of anger and amusement, stopped the show. Finally, came my attorney's closing argument which was short and unexpected. Addressing the jurors, he intelligently and humanly summed up the whole trial, a trial about the dramatic birth of a child who was right there in front of us, nicely dressed, healthy and happy, puzzled as to why he had to be there. "This is all about the money, not justice," were the attorney's last words.

The judge decided to retreat with the jurors, before the sentence. When they came back, we all stood up, remaining somber and anxious, as if a life or death sentence was about to be given out.

I was acquitted unanimously. When we parted, I shook my attorney's hand and thanked him. We already had built a personal relationship. He asked me if I would be the defense expert in another one of the cases he had on his agenda. I refused, and in the end, I gave him one of my poetry books, with a dedication. He looked at the book with utmost surprise.

"Congratulations, doctor! You don't seem to be a poet... When I retire, I might start to paint."

As he was walking away I was thinking: "Just get rid of that yellow pad."

He seemed to be a talented sketcher, a man with a good feeling that in today's world everyone should have a second profession, or at least a nice hobby.

ADRIAN SANGEORZAN graduated from the Medical School at the University of Cluj, Transylvania and worked as a doctor in communist Romania until 1990 when he immigrated to the United States. He lives in New York and works as an obstetrician and gynecologist.

His is the author of the book of memoirs and fiction *Exiled from the Womb — Tales of a Women's Doctor.* He also published volumes of poems: *Over the Lifeline, Tattoos on Marble and The Anatomy of the Moon.* He has several books of short stories and novels: *The Circus in Front of the House, Vitali, The Tap on the Shoulder.* He is co-translator of *Naming the Nameless — An Anthology of Contemporary American Poetry.*

Sangeorzan embodies something that's been missing from the American scene since William Carlos Williams: the poet-doctor—a person who works to heal our all-too-impermanent bodies without sacrificing the sensitivity, intellect and humor that nourish our minds and souls.

Bruce Benderson, Author of User

Sangeorzan, in the tradition, and with the brilliance of Chekhov, weaves his own immigrant experience in these tales of a suspenseful human web. He is a writer for our time who answers the recurring question of American identity with exquisite and persuasive art.

Andrei Codrescu, poet and chronicler of American life

One has to be bold and independent in order to be a writer and to be a surgeon… Adrian Sangeorzan understands intuitively with his heart and talent and that is what he tells his reader in every story. His voice is very strong and genuine. This is not a belle lettre but a real voice talking about real things.

Andrey Gritsman, poet and physician

Made in the USA
Middletown, DE
05 November 2026

36588050R00149